Residential Care for the Elderly

**Recent Titles in
Contributions to the Study of Aging**

Geriatric Medicine in the United States and Great Britain
David K. Carboni

Innovative Aging Programs Abroad: Implications for the United States
Charlotte Nusberg, with Mary Jo Gibson and Sheila Peace

The Extreme Aged in America: A Portrait of an Expanding Population
Ira Rosenwaike, with the assistance of Barbara Logue

Old Age in a Bureaucratic Society: The Elderly, the Experts, and the State in American History
David Van Tassel and Peter N. Stearns, editors

The Aged in Rural America
John A. Krout

Public Policy Opinion and the Elderly, 1952–1978
John E. Tropman

The Mirror of Time: Images of Aging and Dying
Joan M. Boyle and James E. Morriss

North American Elders: United States and Canadian Perspectives
Eloise Rathbone-McCuan and Betty Havens, editors

Hispanic Elderly in Transition: Theory, Research, Policy and Practice
Steven R. Applewhite, editor

Religion, Health, and Aging: A Review and Theoretical Integration
Harold George Koenig, Mona Smiley, and Jo Ann Ploch Gonzales

Philanthropy and Gerontology: The Role of American Foundations
Ann H. L. Sontz

Perceptions of Aging in Literature: A Cross-Cultural Study
Prisca von Dorotka Bagnell and Patricia Spencer Soper, editors

Residential Care for the Elderly

CRITICAL ISSUES IN PUBLIC POLICY

Sharon A. Baggett

CONTRIBUTIONS TO THE STUDY OF AGING, NUMBER 13
Erdman B. Palmore, *Series Adviser*

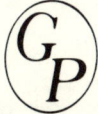

Greenwood Press
NEW YORK • WESTPORT, CONNECTICUT • LONDON

Library of Congress Cataloging-in-Publication Data

Baggett, Sharon.
  Residential care for the elderly : critical issues in public
policy / Sharon A. Baggett.
       p.   cm.— (Contributions to the study of aging, ISSN
0732–085X ; no. 13)
  Bibliography: p.
  Includes index.
  ISBN 0–313–26759–6 (lib. bdg. : alk. paper)
  1. Old age homes—United States. 2. Aged—Institutional care—
Government policy—United States—Evaluation. 3. Old age homes—
Oregon—Case studies. 4. Aged—United States—Functional
assessment. I. Title. II. Series.
HV1461.B34   1989
362.6'1'0973   dc20   89–2152

British Library Cataloguing in Publication Data is available.

Copyright © 1989 by Sharon A. Baggett

All rights reserved. No portion of this book may be
reproduced, by any process or technique, without the
express written consent of the publisher.

Library of Congress Catalog Card Number: 89–2152
ISBN: 0–313–26759–6
ISSN: 0732–085X

First published in 1989

Greenwood Press, Inc.
88 Post Road West, Westport, Connecticut   06881

Printed in the United States of America

The paper used in this book complies with the
Permanent Paper Standard issued by the National
Information Standards Organization (Z39.48–1984).

10 9 8 7 6 5 4 3 2 1

For Lizzie

Contents

Illustrations	ix
Preface	xi
Abbreviations	xiii
Introduction	xv
1. Residential Care: Conceptual Development	1
2. Demand for Residential Care Alternatives	13
3. Supply Factors in Long-Term Care and the Growth of Residential Alternatives	37
4. Development of a Policy Issue and Regulatory Response	53
5. The Oregon Experience	79
6. Characteristics of Residential Care Facility Residents: An Exploratory Analysis	107
7. Relationship Between Regulations/Industry and Needs of Consumers	131
8. Agenda for the Future: A Reformist View	139
References	153
Index	165

Illustrations

FIGURES

3.1	Variability in Market Structure: Nursing Homes and Residential Care	52
4.1	Comparisons/Contrasts: Growth of Regulatory Response in Nursing Homes and Residential Care Facilities	63
6.1	Two-Way Analysis of Variance with Repeated Measures Design	115
6.2	Main Effects with Interactions: Mental Status	123
6.3	Main Effects with Interactions: Instrumental Activities of Daily Living	124
6.4	Main Effects with Interactions: Physical Activities of Daily Living (PADL)	125
6.5	Main Effects with Interactions: Subjective Mental Health	127
6.6	Interaction Effects: Social Support	129

TABLES

3.1	Number of Licensed Adult Residential Care Beds by Type of Facility, 1983	40
6.1	Demographic Analysis of Respondents	112
6.2	Length of Residence in Metropolitan Study Area	116
6.3	Previous Location	117
6.4	Health Indicators	117

6.5	Respondents' Ability to Take Own Medications (Self-Report)	118
6.6	Health Care Utilization by Respondents During Six Months Prior to Initial Interview	118
6.7	Respondents Reporting Adherence to a Special Diet	119
6.8	Respondents' Reported Levels of Incontinence	119
6.9	Types of Assistance Provided to RCF Residents	120
6.10	Primary Diagnoses of RCF Respondents	121
6.11	Analysis of Covariance: Mental Status	122
6.12	Analysis of Covariance: Instrumental Activities of Daily Living	123
6.13	Analysis of Covariance: Physical Activities of Daily Living	125
6.14	Analysis of Covariance: Affect Functioning	126
6.15	Analysis of Covariance: Subjective Physical Health	127
6.16	Analysis of Covariance: Subjective Mental Health	127
6.17	Analysis of Covariance: Social Support	128

Preface

Writing this book has taken me full circle. Almost twenty years ago I was a young social work student working in a state school for the mentally retarded. The facility itself was seen as a model institution, attracting many bright graduate students, innovative psychologists, and community volunteers. One unit, however, was left untouched by the otherwise creative staff. That unit housed the oldest residents. The lack of attention given to these residents and to many of the older mentally retarded adults whom I trained for "community living" sent me to graduate school to specialize in the new field of gerontology. The years since have provided me the opportunity to work with older adults in nursing homes, residential settings, and senior centers and as case-management clients.

My early experiences with deinstitutionalization of the mentally impaired—lack of funding for staff training, inadequate follow-up, and visits to fearful residents in community placements—have been well documented in recent years. The current trends in community alternatives for the elderly—a deinstitutionalization from nursing homes—have yet to attract the same attention. Yet, the potential for less than adequate care seems just as great in these settings, which often house both the mentally impaired and the aged. Alas, I find myself, years later, asking many of the same questions that came to me as a young student.

This book has thus grown from a long interest in the public choices made about the care of those individuals who depend on others for the basic needs of daily life. Along the way, a few individuals have been beacons of light—illuminating the search for answers, challenging me with even harder questions, and setting standards for research that I still strive to attain. First and foremost, I want to thank Cora Martin, who encouraged me to pursue my academic interests and fostered my curiosity in the subject of aging. She, along with Hiram Friedsam and Marvin Ernst, through their fine scholarship and teaching, provided invaluable training in gerontological theory and research. More recently, Sy Adler has been a friend, critic, and guide. He stimulated me to think in new ways and to appreciate the nuances of public policy analysis and supported me when the project seemed overwhelming. And thanks go to my family, friends, and colleagues who listened to my complaints but restrained themselves from asking, "Why are you doing this?"

I have been blessed to know many older people who have taught me a great deal about the human spirit. I give special thanks to the residents who participated in the study described in Chapter 6. They were willing to share their knowledge and feelings with me during the stressful time of their move to the facility. The staff of the Long Term Care Unit of the Oregon Senior Services Division were also extremely helpful and candid in their comments on the long-term care system. A special thanks goes to Lu Dethlefs.

Due to the controversial nature of the role of residential care facilities, the sources of some of the interviews remain anonymous. This should not in any way detract from the usefulness and power of the information.

Finally, immense gratitude to Rob for the music that washed over me throughout this process.

Abbreviations

ADL	Activities of Daily Living
AFS	Adult and Family Services
ANCOVA	Analysis of Covariance
AOA	Administration on Aging
BCCU	Board and Care Coordinating Unit
CCMU	Client Care Monitoring Unit
CON	Certificate of Need
CPI	Consumer Price Index
DHHS	Department of Health and Human Services
DHR	Department of Human Resources
DHUD	Department of Housing and Urban Development
DRG	Diagnosis-Related Groups
GATES	Geriatric Assessment Testing and Evaluation System
HA	Homes for the Aged
HCFA	Health Care Financing Administration
HEW	Health, Education, and Welfare
HI	Health Insurance
HIS	Health Interview Survey
IADL	Instrumental Activities of Daily Living
ICF	Intermediate Care Facility
IG	Inspector General
IHA	Institute for Health and Aging
IRS	Internal Revenue Service
MED	Mentally and Emotionally Disabled

MFI	Master Facilities Inventory
MRDD	Mentally Retarded/Developmentally Disabled
NCHS	National Center for Health Statistics
OAA	Older Americans Act
OBRA	Omnibus Reconciliation Act
OPE	Other Payroll Expenses
OSHD-HFLC	Oregon State Health Department–Health Facilities Licensure and Certification
PADL	Physical Activities of Daily Living
RCF	Residential Care Facility
RCFE	Residential Care Facility for the Elderly
SBA	Small Business Administration
SNF	Skilled Nursing Facility
SOP	Standard Operating Procedure
SPES	Short Psychiatric Evaluation Schedule
SPMSQ	Short Portable Mental Status Questionnaire
SSD	Senior Services Division
SSI	Supplemental Security Income
SSP	State Supplemental Payment
TEFRA	Tax Equity and Fiscal Responsibility Act

Introduction

Recent decades have witnessed the growth of an array of housing and care options for older adults. Specifically, residential care facilities (RCFs) have developed to provide personal care and oversight to older people, the mentally impaired, and the disabled. Currently, RCFs are a major component of the long-term care system in this country. Yet the growth in their numbers has not elicited the attention of policy makers or researchers in long-term care. The term *residential care* actually refers to many different types of housing/care arrangements with great variety in the types and levels of services provided.

To confound understanding of this alternative further, these facilities are referred to by various names in different states. These names include residential care, sheltered care, assisted living, domiciliary care, congregate care, adult foster care, personal care homes, family care, group homes, and homes for the aged (Reichstein & Bergofsky, 1983; Harrington et al., 1985; Mor et al., 1986). As established by state regulations, they provide, at a minimum, room, board, supervision, and protective oversight; in addition they may provide assistance with activities of daily living (for example, bathing, grooming, eating), medication supervision, and in some instances assistance with transportation or obtaining medical and social services (Kochhar, 1977; Harrington et al., 1985; Mor et al., 1986). This range in service provision "makes client identification, regulation and possible reimbursement (especially cost-related reimbursement) very difficult to design and implement" (Palmer, 1983, p. 437). Moreover, even within a given state, the name and regulations governing a residential alternative may vary by kind of population served, number of residents in a specific accommodation, nature of the setting, or number of people per bedroom.

For the purposes of this analysis, residential care in the broad sense includes any facility, operated for profit or otherwise, which accommodates or is designed to accommodate two or more adults unrelated to the owner or operator and which provides room and board on a 24-hour basis to primarily non-transient aged . . . persons who require some personal care, supervision, or assistance in daily activities such as bathing, dressing, or the taking of medicine prescribed for self-administration. (Temple University, 1977, p. 3)

Unless otherwise specified in the following analysis (as in chapters 5 and 6), the term *residential care* is used generically to cover the range of options described above and will be used interchangeably with the term *sheltered* (or *extra-sheltered*) *housing,* which is the term most often used in the literature of Western Europe.

RESEARCH FOCUS

Residential care is growing rapidly as a form of housing and service provision for older adults. The research reported here takes as its premise that RCFs have developed and now deliver a wide array of services in a policy environment of confusion and conflicting directions. The initial chapter describes several policy positions, summarizes the research approaches utilized, and reviews the belief systems that form the background for research in housing and care for older people. The regulatory context in which RCFs operate and the changes in the long-term care system as a whole have contributed to confusion about the appropriate design and use of RCFs. Since RCFs lack a clear role as housing and/or care, a state of indefiniteness exists, in which policy develops without a distinct aim. Residential care policy is thus defined by historical and cultural influences in social policy development and in the regulation of long-term care, specifically for nursing homes. These influences have played a large role in the growing regulatory environment for residential care. Both the realities of the industry and the residents it serves, however, may call for a more creative response—one based on current knowledge and experience rather than on preestablished routines for regulation in housing and health care for the elderly.

In particular, this book examines the characteristics of elderly RCF residents and reviews these through the lens of current state and federal regulations concerning the type of care provided in these facilities. The hypothesis is that the lack of knowledge regarding the characteristics of older persons who choose RCF care promotes facility design and regulations for living environments in which inappropriate care and oversight may be given. That is, there may be a mismatch between the stated purpose of facilities and regulations, on the one hand, and the clients who must be served, on the other.

Within this framework, the policy analysis of residential care consists of two distinct research tasks. The first includes an analysis of both the factors that contribute to the growth of residential care and also the current federal and state policies that define the character of residential alternatives. This review provides a context for examining in some detail actual implementation of these policies. In particular, Oregon's residential care program shows how one state has implemented federal initiatives and defined residential care within the state's goals and philosophies of long-term care. Through a study of the funding mechanisms, regulations, and the role of state agencies in development and monitoring compliance, a detailed picture of residential care in Oregon emerges. Parallels to developments in other states are then drawn.

The second level of research provides information about the characteristics of residential care users. Specifically, data collected from a residential care population and from a sample of older persons in different living environments illustrate the characteristics of older persons residing in one RCF, the services they need to maintain successful residence in the RCF environment, and the ways in which these residents differ from the larger elderly population. A comprehensive functional assessment instrument was used to gather data on the resident and comparison samples; it is introduced as one method that policy makers can use to gather more adequate knowledge regarding users of RCFs.

Finally, the policy context and the quantitative data are linked in a new synthesis. The synthesis sheds light on the role of comprehensive functional assessment in determining which individuals need and use RCFs and on the policy issues implied in the use of such an instrument. It also provides a base for assessing the appropriateness of current RCF regulations and the future of residential care, particularly in Oregon. Such an analysis, linking the larger policy issues with an in-depth analysis of one residential facility's residents and services, should be helpful to policy planners, developers, administrators, and case managers who assist older people with care choices, as well as to older consumers of housing and residential care services.

Residential Care for the Elderly

CHAPTER 1

Residential Care: Conceptual Development

CONCEPTUAL CONFUSION: IS IT HOUSING OR IS IT CARE?

Residential care, in its development as a form of housing and/or service provision for elderly persons, has been caught in a peculiar bind. On the one hand, the framers of policy have tried to retain the noninstitutional character of such residential alternatives. On the other, evidence of abuse (for example, lack of necessary medical care, exploitation, physical abuse) in these facilities and the level of frailty of many residents require that regulations be implemented to assure the quality of care provided. Trying to accomplish these often contradictory goals has left a confusing state, within which the potential for inadequate care is great.

Contributing to this bind is the lack of a clear definition of the role of residential care or other forms of assisted living. The purpose of assisted living may be viewed as twofold. It may provide housing for individuals needing a supervised living situation, in which minimal assistance is provided. Alternatively, sheltered or assisted housing may be a form of care provision itself, in which more extensive medical and personal care assistance is available. Assisted living brings into focus the sometimes conflicting priorities of the social services, housing experts, and health care providers whose emphases in residential care may vary.

In long-term care for the elderly, the roots of the dichotomy between housing and care are similar to the conflicts between the medical and social models of care. The biological and biomedical models of aging have contributed to the perception of old age as an individual problem (physiological decline with chronological age). Aging is thus seen as independent of social structure and as largely a medical problem. This view does not, however, take into account social factors contributing to disease nor the social problems that accompany illness and decline.

This emphasis on the medical model has contributed to the dominance of medical care in the allocation of public resources for the elderly and "has resulted in the medicalization of services, as exemplified in the high proportion of publicly financed health expenditures allocated to hospital and physician coverage, as opposed to community, in-home and other social services" (Estes & Lee, 1985, p. 21). At the same time, the costly nature of long-term care and its perceived lack of professional reward for physicians have focused the health care financing system on acute care for older persons in hospital settings. This financing system is, however, inadequate for providing services for the vast majority of older persons with chronic illnesses, who need supervision or support with the activities of daily living for an extended period of time.

In long-term care, the emphasis on the medical model has directed the bulk of public long-term care resources to the nursing home. As Estes and Lee (1985) have noted:

As de facto long term care policy, nursing homes have been required to perform multiple functions—custodial care, acute illness care, rehabilitation, chronic care, and terminal care—without the resources to perform these tasks.... Alternative policies for the provision of income maintenance, housing, and social supports have not been implemented because the dominant medical model has consumed resources that otherwise could have supported such policies. (pp. 21–22)

Advocates for the elderly have actively lobbied for the inclusion of regulations addressing the social needs of residents in nursing homes and for resources to implement these requirements. The nursing home industry, however, remains dominated by the medical model of care. The extent to which this model may come to dominate the residential care industry is an issue addressed throughout the remainder of this volume.

Recent developments that foster the use of community alternatives to nursing home care have contributed to the confusion regarding the role of the residential care setting. Many states consider residential care a housing expenditure under their federally funded/state-supplemented Supplemental Security Income (SSI) program; changes in other federal legislation also provide for additional care and services to residents of all types of community care dwellings. Thus, Title XX of the Social Security Act, modified and renamed the Social Services Block Grant by the Omnibus Budget Reconciliation Act (OBRA) of 1981, allowed states much more flexibility in using social services funds. Many have used this flexibility to provide support services for community-based elderly, including those in residential care settings. In addition, the 1978 amendments to Title III of the Older Americans Act (OAA) consolidated funds to states for social services and meals and mandated a proportion that must be used for access services (for example, transportation, information, and referral), in-home services, and legal services. Perhaps most important, Section 2176 of OBRA granted the secretary of the Department of Health and Human Services (DHHS) the authority to waive existing Medicaid requirements in order to allow states to use Medicaid funds to finance community-based, noninstitutional care. Allowable services under the waivers included case management, homemaker, home-health aide, personal care, adult day health, rehabilitation, and respite care (Harrington et al., 1985). More recently, Section 4102 of U.S. Public Law 100–203, the Omnibus Reconciliation Act of 1987, continued the Medicaid waiver program and broadened allowable services.

In states where coordination efforts among programs have been attempted, a single elderly person, particularly with low income, may be served by any one or all of these programs. As an example, a case manager may put together a service package that is designed to postpone the institutionalization of a frail older person and that uses SSI funds to pay for board and care, with transportation to medical and social services arranged through OAA-funded programs and case management and home health visits provided through the Medicaid waiver program. This packaging concept, while a positive move toward the coordination of services to meet clients' needs, further blurs the distinction between residential care as a housing option and residential care as one phase of long-term health care.

This confusion in identity only adds to the difficulty encountered by policy makers in designing regulations and considering reimbursement for this type of community support. In Great Britain, for example, this same lack of clarity is cited as a continuing impediment to the evolution of workable financing for sheltered housing; as such, it is identified as a contributor to a less-than-satisfactory relationship between the providers of welfare services and the developers of sheltered housing. This division between welfare and housing services extends to arguments about who should control the allotment of available sheltered housing. Similarly, it extends to which services should reasonably be given over to social service departments and which should be the responsibility of health departments (Butler et al., 1983).

This confusion between merely supervised housing and housing with more extensive medical and personal care has been exacerbated in recent years by several additional factors. First, the aging of the population in existing retirement and board and care facilities has produced debate regarding the amount of care that can reasonably be provided in developments designed primarily as housing for more active older adults. This concern can be seen in both the private sector and in public housing authority programs, including recent longitudinal experiments begun with "service minimal" and "service intensive" congregate housing programs for the elderly (Byerts & Heller, 1985). In England, this same concern is reflected in the call for "very sheltered housing" for those older people reaching advanced age in existing sheltered housing units. Second, a shortage of institutional beds and changes in the delivery of health care have contributed to a more frail, more dependent elderly population returning to other community care options, such as retirement apartments, primarily designed to provide shelter, not care.

The impact of these factors can readily be seen in the emerging physical design requirements for residential facilities. Newer buildings may more closely resemble the institutions they were designed to replace. In some facilities, the option to purchase "extra care" may render them a near match with nursing homes. With increasing recognition that residential care of this intensity may also require much more extensive funding to assure the quality and quantity of care come calls for federal reimbursement. As the residential care industry develops, clarification of the housing versus care issue will become increasingly important. Perhaps the argument most clearly emerges as how much care can be provided in the various housing/care options currently available, and do current policies and regulations reflect these realities? It is also necessary to examine the likely outcomes if either model—housing or care—should predominate. Basically, the housing model assumes an active, independent population in need of minimal assistance. The care model assumes a level of frailty among residents requiring a great deal of supportive services and medical (primarily nursing) intervention. Acceptance of the housing model seems unlikely to continue, as residential alternatives are increasingly used to provide care for an older, sicker population. The predominance of the health care model for residential facilities, however, will have tremendous implications for cost, reimbursement, regulation, and the vision of residential care as a nonmedical, noninstitutional alternative.

The focus, regardless of the model, needs to be clarified. The ongoing ideal of the housing model, preferred for its positive philosophical goal of community care, combined with the reality of the medical care model's growth, leaves a confusing milieu in which to define policy and insure quality of support, whatever the environment.

Yet there is also danger in seeing the residential care issue as a dichotomy, for, in reality, the social, housing, and medical care needs of older people overlap. The dominance of the medical model could result in the residential industry more closely resembling the nursing home industry, as stated earlier, with the potential for ignoring the needs of residents in terms of privacy, self-determination, and social/psychological support. To ignore the increasing medical needs and particularly the mental health needs of the frail population in residential facilities would also be unacceptable. Current policies have not addressed these crucial issues. Before an analysis of such policies can be undertaken, a review of the development of the concept of residential care is necessary.

CONCEPTUAL DEVELOPMENT OF RESIDENTIAL CARE: FACTORS, DEFINITIONS, RATIONALES

Factors

The general consensus framing many of the services designed for the elderly appears to be that people become frail and debilitated as they age; in the normal course of aging, they reach some critical point beyond which they are no longer able to care for themselves completely. After reaching this stage, they must depend on others for some support and assistance, whether in their own homes or in protective settings. "This model is essentially the underpinning of both the nursing home industry and the Older Americans Act [cf. Estes, 1979] and has been characterized [Zarit, 1980] as the philosophy of custodialism" (Knight & Walker, 1985). Indeed, in the field of human services, few topics have received as much attention in recent years as has the care of frail older people in our society. This group, the old old, "consists of persons, usually but not always, over the age of 75, who because of the accumulation of various continuing problems often require one or several supportive services in order to cope with daily life" (DHEW, 1978a, p. 1).

In response to the growth of this population, substantial effort has been expended on designing services and care options that would be responsive to the needs of a potentially large, although not well-defined, client population. This population has been the focus of the development of a "long-term-care system," and people are generally thought to need long-term care "when they have a chronic disease or condition which causes both functional impairment and physical dependence on others . . . a situation referred to as functional disability" (DHHS, 1981b, p. 3).

Subsequently, housing and care options have developed to meet the needs of older persons as they reach various stages of dependency, the so-called "continuum of care" (Hillhaven Foundation, 1980). Inherent in this model is the concept of movement along the continuum, with increasingly intensive and costly service needed as the older individual becomes more frail. Knight and Walker (1985) have acknowledged that "there is a tendency to assume that the elderly decline in some progressive way and move up through the range of institutions as they deteriorate" (p. 360).

In part as a result of these beliefs, a range of housing and service options for older adults has developed in recent decades. These options have also increasingly been advocated as alternatives for support and care for those elderly and mentally impaired who do not need institutionalization or the extensive nursing care provided in nursing homes. Moreover, the perception of nursing homes as places fraught with abuse, as dehumanizing environments for older people, and as an expensive form of care based on the medical model has also led to a search for alternatives. In addition to nursing home care and home delivery of health services, options have developed that might be called "assisted living" or "sheltered care," that is, congregate living with supportive services provided on-site.

Definitions

As noted, residential care facilities developed in response to a need for personal care and oversight for older people, the mentally impaired, and the disabled.

The term has now come to represent a broad array of alternatives within the long-term care continuum. Before the recent advent of Medicaid, homes of all types served the dependent population of aged. The introduction of Medicaid nursing home reimbursement forced a distinction between homes providing personal care but nonmedical treatment to the aged and those providing medical support. It also imposed licensure or certification requirements for facilities in these distinct categories. As Sherwood et al. (1980) found, any home desiring Medicaid certification was required to meet strict guidelines governing physical plant, personnel regulations, and patient care. Following the separation of skilled nursing facilities (SNFs) from other types of nursing facilities, additional regulatory guidelines were sought to distinguish board and care homes from nursing homes (Palmer, 1983). Some of these homes eventually became nursing homes, while others became residential care facilities.

In the past, these homes served the mentally ill, developmentally disabled, and, more recently, the aged. Unfortunately, while a substantial literature describes homes serving the mentally ill and disabled (Gollay et al., 1978; Melick & Eysaman, 1978; Segal & Aviram, 1978), little is known about residential facilities serving the aged, their growth over the past decades, or the aged residents of these facilities. Several factors have inhibited research in this field. These include the changes in the industry following the Medicaid legislation and the "semantic tangle" (Palmer, 1983) caused by the different states' names and definitions of facilities. Further, it is difficult to delineate the numerous agencies involved in oversight of these facilities. Indeed, in their survey of the states, Mor et al. (1986) identified 118 residential programs with twenty-one different names. Most programs were under the supervision of several regulatory agencies.

Before a further review of the residential care industry and the policies that have shaped its character, it is crucial to examine the cultural beliefs and professional ideologies that shape the theory underlying this type of care. As Estes (1979) has noted, while empirical research provides a partial basis for policy development in care for the aged, "even more important is the potential contribution of gerontological theory to the underlying rationale for those policies" (p. 7).

Theories, Assumptions, and Rationales

Services in the United States that have developed to meet the needs of older people imply a continuum of age-related deterioration (individual processes). The service system is seen as a combination of environmental factors that can be altered to adapt to these changes within older people. This view of old age and the surrounding social system reflects the predominant theoretical approach of symbolic interactionism among American gerontologists. They tend to examine problems in terms of the individual and his or her adjustment to the wider social circumstances. This view of aging, drawing on a number of empirical studies (Rose & Peterson, 1965; Trela, 1971; Gubrium, 1973; Hendricks &

Henricks, 1977), has argued "that it is possible for the interactional context and process (the environment, the persons, and encounters in it) to significantly affect the kind of aging process a person will experience" (Estes, 1979, p. 9).

This theoretical framework focuses on both environment and the individual. One policy response expected would therefore be interventions that attempt to modify environmental variables (type of housing, elimination of age discrimination, and promotion of age differentiation). Another response would be directed to the needs of the individual aging person, such as improved health care through Medicare and meals programs. Butler et al. (1983) asserted that sheltered housing programs, both in the United States and Great Britain, have been based on this theoretical underpinning, with its focus on an individualistic form of explanation; the rationale for the development of the programs is based on assumptions growing out of this theoretical premise. Reliance on this rationale results in a great faith in the "social engineering of old age" on the part of sheltered housing advocates (Butler et al., 1983, p. 37). That is, there is "a belief that changing the type of accommodation an old person inhabits will in some way result in a richer social life, less feelings of social isolation, and the prolongation of active life" (Underwood & Carver, 1979, p. 78).

Proponents of sheltered housing for the elderly offer a variety of rationales for its development based on the belief system described above. While presented separately, they are interrelated and have an impact on design, management, targeted population, public policy, and regulation. The rationales identified by Butler et al. (1983) and others (Dalley, 1988) include:

Need for Appropriate Housing. The first rationale offered for providing specialized housing is that many older people currently live in inadequate or unsuitable housing. This may include housing that is too large or under-occupied. That is, the older person now occupies a large home that once provided room for children and extended family. A reduced income may make heating and other maintenance of a large dwelling financially prohibitive. In other cases, existing housing may be substandard. That is, the home may lack standard amenities, be difficult to adapt for special needs, or be unsafe from an inspector's view when the older adult develops new safety needs. While little empirical evidence has been provided to justify building specialized housing versus investing in home improvement, adapting existing housing to smaller family size, or simply moving individuals into better quality housing, the bias toward sheltered housing still exists. In other countries, such as England, this bias may be fed by the additional pressure of scarce housing, which increases the demand that older people relinquish underoccupied houses to provide housing stock for younger families.

Special Needs. Another underlying rationale for sheltered housing portrays older people as a special group within society who must be treated differently and provided with specially designed services and living quarters. This view may be based on the premise that many older people have disabilities that require specially designed housing features. The assumption is made as well that older people may be viewed as a cohesive group, with similar tastes and requirements, including the need for economical cooking, heating, and living space. These beliefs are often reflected in the actual design of environments, with many facilities providing little storage, and small one-bedroom or studio apartments, kitchenettes, or no cooking facilities at all. A curious contradiction in this belief system can be seen in the popular notions that (1) older people desire a peaceful, idyllic view from their domicile, yet (2) older people are bored and lonely and need to see activity from the windows of their dwelling. These beliefs, fostered by younger designers, assume a certain level of passivity among the elderly (Townsend, 1981) and deny the variety of personal styles and tastes of the heterogeneous elderly population. If we examine the variety of housing options available for all other age groups, there is no empirical evidence to suggest that the same variety of housing choice is not desired by older persons.

The harshest critics of the trend toward segregated, specialized housing for older people warn of the dangers of stigmatizing and disabling the very population the policy intends to serve. They point to trends in other areas of social policy away from special provision in segregated settings and toward incorporation of these groups into the mainstream (such as educational provision for the mentally and physically handicapped) (Tinker, 1977a). It seems realistic, however, to assume that some older people may need or desire special housing. It should perhaps be only one alternative in an array of possible accommodations, where the primary focus is on providing adequate supports to allow older persons to continue their home life in normal surroundings. Interestingly, the adult foster home or small board and care facility appears to be an attempt to provide a hybrid alternative, where special provision for care is made in a more natural and home-like environment rather than in a large, institutional setting.

Choice. The development of sheltered housing and other forms of special housing for older persons has been seen as progress in offering them a wider range of choices about where to live. Making an educated choice, however, assumes knowledge about the range of services offered. While little research exists regarding the extent to which older people or their families are aware of the options available to them, development continues under the assumption that many older people would choose specially designed accommodations. The fact that until recently little private development has occurred in this area may also indicate a lack of desire or demand on the part of older people. When residential care is chosen, it might be posited that, while not ideal, an older person under pressure to move from family, friends, or professional service providers would find this housing acceptable simply because of a fear of more restrictive alternatives such as a nursing home.

Emergency. The thought of an emergency evokes powerful feelings. The image of an older person lying alone on the floor, undiscovered for days and unable to summon help, has been a commanding argument used both by professionals and by families to emphasize the security offered by sheltered housing. While this image is common in the marketing literature for such facilities, there is little empirical evidence about the effectiveness of using alarms to avert emergencies or having twenty-four-hour supervision to cope with emergencies. It appears that we need better assessment mechanisms for measuring the hazards and strengths of a given older person's environment and for assessing his or her physiological and mental capacities so that the risks involved in remaining in a given setting can be more accurately evaluated. Even then, many older people may be comfortable with the image of dying alone and may, if given the option, choose the risk of an unforeseen emergency as a tradeoff for remaining in a familiar environment. For others, the psychological reassurance of having help available if needed may weigh in favor of specialized housing programs.

Loneliness. An interest in the idea of loneliness among the elderly was created in the 1960s, based on the writings of several authors (Townsend, 1962; Tunstall, 1966). Subsequent authors have criticized this work for equating the status of living alone with the subjective state of loneliness (Johnson, 1976). The notion of widespread loneliness in old age was also fed by the now suspect notion of the breakdown of family support for elders (Shanas, 1979); it has generated in turn an abundance of research reporting the support available in existing social networks (Moroney, 1976; Cantor, 1979; Stoller & Stoller, 1983). While evidence has been produced to substantiate the idea that some elderly do feel lonely and isolated (Abrams, 1978; Lowenthal, 1964; Lowenthal & Robinson, 1977), it must be asked whether this incidence is more prevalent than in the population at large and whether options exist for addressing it that do not involve specialized housing schemes. Some limited research has also suggested that segregated, sheltered housing may not be very successful in addressing the needs of the lonely (Page & Muir, 1971). This finding may be viewed with some caution and may simply imply that "those who live alone are not necessarily lonely. ... It seems likely that after years of semi-solitary living they might not take to the inevitably artificial sociability of a sheltered housing scheme" (Butler et al., 1983, p. 47).

In addition, some older persons who relocate to an adult foster care home, usually in a small family-type setting, may have difficulty adjusting to such intimacy after living alone and may feel pressure to socialize with strangers, thus actually increasing feelings of isolation. Perhaps equally important is the fact that the level of frailty of those occupying sheltered housing, particularly a high level of sensory and/or mental impairment, may make resocialization extremely difficult regardless of the setting.

Community Care. A dominant premise has been that the goal is alternatives to institutional care, with the underlying belief that community care (particularly care within one's own home) is inherently more satisfying, more natural, and less costly. The denigration of institutional care has grown out of a literature citing the dehumanizing and often abusive aspects of life in a nursing home or similar institution (Goffman, 1961; Townsend, 1962; Henry, 1963; Gubrium, 1975; Mendelson, 1974; Moss & Halamandaris, 1977). Public policy for the elderly and the mentally impaired has thus rallied behind the goal of keeping people active and independent in their own homes or, in the case of sheltered housing, keeping them in a "less-restrictive" environment that more closely approximates living in one's own home. These policies are based on

> a normative framework of "family care as best." ... In recent years there has been a publicly achieved consensus between policy makers, practitioners and "experts" from the academic world that the family model of care is the appropriate policy goal, and it is one which should be applied in all fields of dependency. It has figured prominently in the deinstitutionalisation debate, so that the revulsion rightly felt towards the grossest examples of dehumanised institutional care has been directly linked with the view that the appropriate alternative in all cases is family-based care. Where that form of care is not available, then measures which are "nearest approximations to that form" are introduced. (Dalley, 1988, p. 25).

Ironically, the assumption is also made that it is more efficient and cost-effective to deliver services to concentrated, homogeneous populations such as those in larger residential care facilities. The irony is that the opposite argument, that is, that it is more cost-effective to keep older persons in their own homes, has also been used to defend community alternatives to care such as home health services. These services have been advocated as a less costly substitute for nursing home care and as a mechanism for postponing institutionalization.

While increasing effort has focused on evaluating the effectiveness of alternative forms of care, including cost-effectiveness (Stassen & Holahan, 1981; Packwood, 1981), this work is inconclusive. Convincing documentation that community alternatives clearly improve the quality of life, postpone institutionalization, or are cost-effective or cheaper than institutional care has yet to be produced. Butler et al. (1983) have pointed out that, in addition to the lack of conclusive research, the term *community care* "carries with it implications of warmth, concern and altruism, such that it becomes almost reprehensible to question some of its premises.... It may be that it is not institutional care per se which is damaging [or inferior], but simply impoverished care of any kind" (p. 49). Thus, policy that fosters the development of alternatives to institutional care and that is based on a belief in their inherent superiority without concern for adequate financial reimbursement to insure the quality of these alternatives may not contribute to positive options for housing and care.

Independence. The concept of independence appears throughout the literature on housing alternatives. While the concept is rarely defined, it has alternately referred to independence in maintaining one's own dwelling, independence in housekeeping, or merely the psychological perception of independence. In an evaluation of the effectiveness of residential care options in achieving this objective—independence—part of the difficulty lies in defining and measuring the concept. In addition, existing research challenges the belief that sheltered housing contributes to independence (Gray, 1976, 1977) and argues that it may in fact create greater dependency in older people. In addition, Bytheway and James (1978) note that much of residential care/sheltered housing is starting to resemble a "quasi-institution" and appears more and more like a nursing home. This particular tendency will be discussed more fully as the impact of policy and regulation in the fields of long-term care and residential care is reviewed.

REVIEW

In summary, both the history of care for the aged and the dependent and our beliefs about the role of environment in meeting their needs have shaped the policies defining housing and care alternatives. In particular, residential care has grown in response to both deeply held beliefs regarding the type of care that is most suitable and also the historical development of its counterpart, the nursing home. It should be clear from this review that this form of housing is likely to continue to play an important role in housing for the dependent elderly and the disabled in the future and that discussion regarding the type of support it provides will also continue.

CHAPTER 2

Demand for Residential Care Alternatives

The current level of interest in residential care alternatives grows out of several factors. These include the philosophical beliefs regarding community alternatives to institutional care discussed above as well as the social and economic factors that contribute to the demand for such alternatives. These can be divided into two categories of demand factors.

The first are those factors that emerge from population characteristics and include changing demographic trends and the prevalence of frailty or need for service within the population. The dramatic growth of the elderly population in general is a major factor in the demand for care and services of many types. Moreover, the increasing number of frail and/or disabled older adults further intensifies the need for health and welfare services among those in need of long-term care.

The second category of factors includes those political and economic forces that generate demand for particular health and service delivery systems. The rapidly changing nature of the health care system and particularly the rising cost of health services are perhaps the most critical of these forces in determining the demand for long-term care options at this time. An understanding of these demand factors and their interrelated nature is important in order to analyze more fully the ways in which they have shaped policy responses in the long-term care continuum and especially in the emerging residential care industry.

DEMAND FACTORS: POPULATION CHARACTERISTICS

Demographics

America's older population is larger than it has ever been and, if current trends persist, the number of older persons will continue to grow into the next century.

Three aspects of the growth of this population contribute to this trend: (1) the absolute number of older people in the population and their characteristics; (2) the proportion of the total population who are elderly; and (3) the longevity of given individuals, as seen in changing life expectancy figures. Primarily because of a combination of high birthrates during the early part of the twentieth century and long-term decline in mortality rates, the rapid growth of the elderly population is largely a phenomenon of this century. In 1900, for example, only about 4 percent of the population was over 65 years of age. By 1940, persons aged 65 and over totaled about 9 million and comprised about 6.8 percent of the total population. The elderly had grown to over 9 percent by 1960, and in 1980 there were 25.9 million persons aged 65 and over, comprising almost 11.1 percent of the total population of 233 million (Rice & Feldman, 1983; Zopf, 1986). It is of special interest that since 1960 the elderly have grown in number more than twice as fast as all younger population groups. Current estimates project that between 1980 and 2040 the total population will grow by 41 percent, while the elderly population will double to a total of 55 million, or 22 percent of the population (Rice & Feldman, 1983).

The increased number of the very old, or the so-called "fourth generation," is perhaps a still more critical trend in any analysis of long-term care issues. The concept of the fourth generation refers to the growth in the population of persons over 75 years of age and can be "attributed to not only greater longevity but also to earlier marriages and earlier childbearing, which reduces the average span in years between generations" (Estes & Lee, 1985, p. 25). This population is growing even more rapidly than the elderly population as a whole. Thus, while the elderly population as a whole grew from 9.1 percent to 11.1 percent of the total population from 1960 to 1980, in the same time span those aged 75 to 84 grew 65 percent while those 85 years and over increased 174 percent. By the year 2000, those 75 and over are expected to increase from 38 percent of the current elderly population to 45 percent (Rice & Feldman, 1983).

The growth of the fourth generation can be seen as an example of the significant social changes that have occurred in this century. These changes can be expected to continue. The majority of this group, the old old, are women, primarily unmarried or widowed. They are likely to have significant levels of functional impairment, higher rates of health care utilization than younger age groups, and fewer resources with which to meet economic and social needs. Additional demographic trends, such as the decline or leveling off of the birthrate and the increasing participation of women in the work force, may reduce the availability of the family as the primary provider of personal care for older persons needing assistance (Brody et al., 1983; Brody & Schoonover, 1986).

Several major trends that now shape the profile of the aging population will also affect populations of the future. First, life expectancy at birth, which has increased by about nine years for males and twelve years for females since 1940, may continue to increase in the coming decades. There is general agreement that life expectancy for the species is limited (somewhere around 100 years), and the trend described here does not imply extending this limit. Rather, it describes the reality of a larger number of people who now live much closer to this limit.

Second, the nation's birthrate, while high during the boom following World War II, fell during the 1960s and has now leveled off at about 1.85 births per woman. If projections that the birthrate will rise only to replacement level (2.1 children for each woman by the 1990s) are accurate, and if this trend persists into the early years of the twenty-first century, the elderly will continue to grow as a share of the total population.

Third, the baby boom of 1945–60 will swell the ranks of the elderly in the years after 2010, and those retiring in the coming decades may do so earlier. They will thereby place increasing demands on the economic support system already strained by a growing retired population, inflation, and other economic factors.

All of these trends raise difficult questions not only about the economic effects of supporting an increasingly large, nonworking population, but also about the effects on health and welfare services. These trends also raise questions about the family and its ability to care for elderly members and about effects on the social and political system, which must respond to the needs of the population as a whole.

Population Characteristics

Health Status. In addition to the social characteristics of the population, such as the large proportion of women, the unmarried, and the widowed among the elderly, the health status of older persons differs perceptibly from that of younger people. In particular, the presence of chronic and disabling disease is a critical factor in analyzing the impact of the growing elderly population. As Rice and Feldman (1983) have indicated: "There are now many more persons suffering from conditions that are managed or controlled rather than cured. These conditions cause afflictions for decades, impairing ability to function and requiring much medical care" (p. 363). This trend produces an increase in the demand for health services at a time when the costs of medical care are rising. Yet limited information is available on the incidence of functional impairment or on its impact on support services across the age spectrum.

The most frequent chronic health conditions reported by the elderly are multiple types of heart disease, hypertension (high blood pressure), and arthritis (Eustis et al., 1984). Those conditions reported as the main cause for limiting activity include heart disease, arthritis, and chronic rheumatism (Butler & Newacheck, 1981). While not all chronic conditions are associated with disability or functional impairment, the incidence of disabling conditions is much higher for the elderly than for others.

One of the few sources for estimating disability, and thus the potential need for long-term care services, is the nationwide Health Interview Survey (HIS), conducted annually by the National Center for Health Statistics. The survey collects data on three related measures: the presence of a chronic disease or condition; limitations in mobility and/or usual activity; and the need of assistance in basic activities in daily living (ADL) such as bathing, dressing, eating, and going to the toilet. From these data, one can extrapolate to those needing care and support services. In 1981, 32 million people (14 percent of the noninstitutionalized population) were estimated to suffer some degree of activity limitation due to a chronic condition, and 3.6 percent of these people were unable to carry out their major daily activities. With age, the prevalence of limitation rose dramatically, with the elderly four and one-half times more likely to suffer limitations of activity compared to the nonelderly. Statistics showed that 14.4 percent of those between 65 and 74, 22.0 percent of those between 75 and 84, and 32.9 percent of those 85 years of age and over were unable to carry out their major activities of daily living. Of those needing personal care assistance in ADL, persons over age 75 were twenty times more likely to need assistance in at least one of the four basic activities than were those under age 65 (U.S. DHHS, 1981b, pp. 5, 6). The impact of these limitations was also reported by Feller (1983), who found that, among the noninstitutionalized population in 1979, 5 percent of those 65–74 years of age, compared with 35 percent of those 85 years and over, needed help in one or more of the major activities of daily living.

These figures are striking when viewed in conjunction with the growth of the population. In the 1980 national HIS, 3.1 million noninstitutionalized persons were reported needing assistance in one or more ADL. By 2040, this number is expected to more than double, to about 7.9 million persons, while the population as a whole is expected to increase by only two-fifths (Rice & Feldman, 1983, p. 377). This difference can be attributed to the aging of the population and is shown even more clearly by the change in distribution by age. That is, "in 1980, 36 percent of noninstitutionalized persons with limitations in ADL were aged 75 and over; by 2040, the proportion rises to 58 percent" (Rice & Feldman, 1983, p. 377). From a slightly different perspective, Kane and Kane (1981) estimated that for every nursing home resident there are three elderly people of equal functional impairment living in the community.

Other demographic factors affecting the incidence of functional impairment among the elderly include income, sex, and race. Butler and Newacheck (1981) found that older persons with annual incomes below $5000 had a greater proportion of major activity limitation than those with higher incomes. They note that this in turn limited their flexibility in choosing and purchasing long-term care services. Elderly males generally exhibit a higher prevalence of major activity limitation than do females—44 percent of males (4 million) compared to 35 percent of females (4.5 million), particularly in the young old, although this difference all but disappears among those of very advanced age. Elderly women in general, however, have a greater chance of being institutionalized than elderly men. Elderly nonwhites in all age categories have greater functional impairment levels than whites; this difference increases with advancing age.

The impact of these levels of impairment on long-term care is visible. Eustis et al. (1984), in estimating supply and demand for the calendar year 1976 (using a variety of federal data sources), reported total long-term care demand at 5.5 to 5.9 million adults, with 0.1 to 0.6 million in need of personal care or sheltered living environments. Combining all those served in noninstitutional settings, including personal care or domiciliary care, sheltered living arrangements, home care, and adult day care indicates that an estimated 0.5 to 1.3 million disabled adults were served in 1976. This demand should increase as those of the fourth generation continue to age and experience increased levels of impairment.

Some caution is in order, however, in estimating potential demand for services from these data on disability, particularly the demand for noninstitutional services. Much of what we know about the elderly who require assistance or some form of long-term care consists of information that has typically been obtained from the institutionalized population. An understanding of our current system and our planning for the future are substantially constrained by lack of data on the number and characteristics of persons who receive informal care and of consumers of care in noninstitutional settings. Where data exist, they are difficult to combine or interpret. This difficulty derives from the diversity of financing, of service providers, and of service and cost definitions, as well as the variety of assessment techniques for measuring impairment. Further barriers to interpreting existing research include varying program criteria, reporting categories and requirements, and little or no consensus or definitions of disability or need for long-term care. (U.S. Congressional Budget Office, 1977; U.S. GAO, 1981). This lack of information is especially noticeable in the field of residential care.

Mental health status is another critical factor in assessing the ability of older people, particularly the very old, to maintain themselves in an independent living environment. Data on the prevalence of mental health problems among the noninstitutionalized elderly are extremely limited. Estimates of symptoms associated with mental illness vary from 15 to 25 percent among the noninstitutionalized older population. About 10 percent have clinically diagnosed depression, with another 5 to 6 percent exhibiting some form of dementia (U.S. DHHS, FCOA, 1981a). While some limited research has compared the noninstitutionalized population to the nursing home population, the research is inconclusive (see Characteristics of Potential Residential Care Consumers later in this chapter). It is also unclear whether impairment leads to institutionalization or to the use of other supervision or whether impairment occurs following a housing or institutional placement.

Health Care Utilization. The types of illnesses suffered by older persons and their ways of using the health care system are important in assessing the use of long-term care services. In particular, recent changes in the health care system have made the elderly population's use of hospital and physician services increasingly significant. Since older people suffer more chronic and disabling medical conditions compared to younger people, their patterns of medical care utilization reflect their poorer health status. They visit physicians, use hospital and nursing home beds, and utilize home health visits more frequently than the younger population.

Recent estimates from the national HIS reveal that in 1981 those elderly residing in the community had contact with a physician (hospital visits to in-patients excluded) an average of 6.3 times per year, in contrast to an average of 5.1 times for persons aged 45–64. Those elderly with chronic activity limitation, such as those in residential care settings, had even higher rates of contact, with 8.7 visits to physicians per year in contrast to 4.3 visits for persons with no activity limitation (U.S. NCHS, 1981a; U.S. NCHS, 1982a). The majority of these visits occur in physicians' offices. These visits vary slightly by race, with black elderly persons visiting physicians at a rate of 6.6 visits per year compared to 6.4 visits for whites. These rates of visits to physicians also vary by income, with the poorest elderly (those with annual incomes of less than $5,000) reporting 6.7 visits per year versus 6.1 visits per year for those with annual incomes between $5,000–$9,000 (U.S. NCHS, 1983). Such physician visits are also projected to increase by approximately 40 percent, or 60 million visits, by the year 2000, with 74 percent of this increase attributed to the 75 and over age group (U.S. NCHS, 1982b).

Elderly people are hospitalized almost twice as frequently as younger people, and their hospital stays are about 50 percent longer. These trends have been increasing with time. From 1967 to 1980, inpatient days per 1,000 population decreased 6 percent for persons under 65 but increased 6 percent for the elderly (Brody & Persily, 1984). In 1981, the elderly, while comprising 11 percent of the total population, consumed 29.8 percent of hospital short-stay days (U.S. NCHS, 1982a). This use rate is particularly high for the very old. Thus, "only 4 percent of the people were 75 years of age or older in 1981, yet they accounted for 13 percent of the discharges and 21 percent of all the days of care" (Harrington et al., 1985, p. 47).

The elderly, compared to the nonelderly, also use more outpatient hospital services, principally for pathology, radiology, and laboratory services. A recent five-year period saw their use increase by 21 percent (Brody & Persily, 1984). The following description from Brody and Persily emphasized the role played by community hospitals in serving the elderly:

More than 4 million persons aged 65 and over . . . use inpatient facilities at least once a year, . . . outpatient utilization is even more impressive. About 5.5 million older people (almost 25 percent of the aged) receive at least one outpatient service a year, visiting the hospital more than 10 million times for these various medical services. Counting both inpatient admissions and outpatient services, the community general hospital serves the elderly directly for about 20 million episodes each year. (P. 35).

Chronic disease is also reflected in the number of return visits by older persons, with 27 percent of those aged persons admitted to a hospital in a given year returning twice or more in the ensuing year. Hospitalization of the elderly derives from those conditions cited most frequently as health problems, including heart disease, cancer, and stroke, with these diagnoses accounting for 34 percent of the total hospital discharges for those 65 and over (Rice, 1985). In addition to hospital care, the elderly are the primary consumers of long-term nursing home care. While only a small proportion of all the elderly, about 5 percent, are in nursing homes, almost 22 percent of those over 85 are nursing home residents (U.S. NCHS, 1981b). The characteristics of these residents are important to any discussion of residential care, since the users of both care settings increasingly resemble one another.

Residents of nursing homes are primarily white, widowed (69 percent), and female (75 percent), with an average age of 83. Some 40 percent come to the nursing home from their own homes, with another 34 percent coming directly from hospitals. The remainder are transfers from other nursing or mental health facilities (Brody & Persily, 1984). Residents of nursing homes most commonly suffer from hardening of the arteries, senility or dementia, stroke, or mental disorders, and most suffer from multiple chronic conditions, such as heart disease, diabetes, and aftereffects of fractures.

Brody and Persily (1984) have offered an interesting analysis of nursing home use, challenging the belief that most nursing home residents are long-term residents. They estimated that about half of those admitted to skilled nursing facilities (SNFs) are discharged within three months. The short-stay consumers, predominantly male, married, and the younger old, average 1.8 months in the SNF, and over half are private-pay residents. These short-stay residents come primarily from hospitals, and 41 percent return to a private residence. The long-stay group (averaging 2.5 years and more likely to die while in residence) represent largely the old old, female population with lower incomes, many more of whom are supported by Medicaid. Liu and Palesch (1981) reported that the presence of short-stay patients is not accurately documented in the cross-sectional surveys ordinarily used to measure nursing home use. Especially for a discussion of care alternatives, this population may be an important element. That is, they may require personal care assistance or supervision in a protective setting following discharge from a nursing home. While the 41 percent who return home may require home health assistance, the remaining numbers may be suitable candidates for sheltered care settings.

The elderly are also the primary consumers of home health services. In 1977, about 800,000 Medicare beneficiaries received services. Under changes in the Medicaid provisions, this number has increased substantially in the past several years. More than half of those served were over 75 years of age, and most lived in urban areas (Brody & Persily, 1984).

The evidence provided by the data points to rapid growth in demand for health and support services of all kinds. In particular, the demand for home health services and other residential alternatives seems great. For example, research indicates that some nursing home patients do not need the level of care received in an institutional setting and could well be served by home health and social service agencies. Concomitantly, many community-dwelling elderly are not receiving needed long-term care services (Harrington et al., 1985). This fact does not mean that nursing home or hospital utilization will decrease. Rather, it implies that other alternatives should be available to make the most efficient use of health care resources and provide a higher quality of life for recipients.

Characteristics of Potential Residential Care Consumers

Many of the 95 percent of the elderly outside institutions who might potentially choose residential care cannot maintain a totally independent existence. Research on users of noninstitutional care often focuses on home health, homemaker, personal care, and chore services. The users of such services are more likely to be low income and to use publicly supported home care services. This focus is due in large part to program eligibility criteria, and to the fact that the bulk of federal research in this area has focused on Medicare/Medicaid recipients (Barney, 1973).

Additional information on current long-term care users is provided by a Minnesota study (Anderson, Patten, & Greenberg, 1980) comparing older (60+ years) home care and nursing home clients. Compared to the general older population in Minnesota, the home care clients were more likely to be female, unmarried or widowed, and living alone. Compared to nursing home residents, however, home care clients tended to be younger (average 76 versus 82 years) and more likely to be female and married. In addressing functional capacity, the same study found the home care clients to be somewhat incapacitated in areas of mobility and physical self-care but less incapacitated than their counterparts in nursing homes (although there was not so great a difference as might be expected). In addition, the home care clients had overall greater functional incapacity on most dimensions than the intermediate care nursing home clients but were considerably less impaired in mental functioning than the skilled nursing care nursing home residents and somewhat less mentally impaired than the intermediate care residents.

Some research has also been directed toward identifying the characteristics of adult day-care users. Weissert (1978) compared two models of adult day-care (one hospital-based and one a multipurpose model) with two levels of nursing home care. These data on functional capacity suggest that in areas such as walking, toileting, eating, continence, and behavior, the participants in the two day-care models were generally less disabled than their counterparts in the nursing home, and to some extent they had different types of impairments. This finding might be expected, given the continuum of care model presented in the previous chapter.

Little research describes the characteristics of older persons in residential homes. Existing research suffers from limited samples (often state-specific), which reduce their generalizability across states (Newcomer & Grant, 1988). Other studies, such as that done by the Comptroller General's Office (U.S. GAO,

1979) and replicated by Eckert, Namazi, and Kahana (1987), used SSI recipient records to identify boarding homes. One study found that residents of congregate housing, when compared to the rest of the United States elderly population, were more likely to be older, female, single or widowed, white, unemployed, and with annual incomes over $6,000. In addition, congregate housing has tended to have a high proportion of older elderly, a finding that indicates that such housing facilities are a place in which one grows old (U.S. DHUD, 1976).

Other descriptive research has found residential care residents to be the very old, with some studies reporting nearly 30 percent of elderly residents over 80 years of age (Bradshaw et al., 1976; Newman & Sherman, 1977; Watt, 1970). They are also primarily female, sometimes up to approximately 70 percent (Bradshaw et al., 1976; Risdorfer et al., 1971). Gioglio and Jacobsen (1984) examined the health and functional status of client groups in residential facilities in New Jersey. They found that one-half of all residents needed assistance with activities of daily living, and 37 percent of the RCF sample needed some form of mental health services.

A recent article by Mor et al. (1986) is one of very few that attempted to define the scope of residential care and to determine in more detail some of the characteristics of the elderly residing in these facilities. In their survey of 670 residents in six states, they found a similar pattern, with 66 percent of respondents female and 40 percent of respondents over the age of 75. The majority of respondents were widowed. At least one-third scored in the impaired region of the mental status questionnaire.

This review has shown that a striking growth has occurred in the number of older persons in need of personal and medical care. While some research exists on the characteristics of elderly persons using day care, home health services, and nursing homes, very little research has focused on older persons in residential care facilities. Comparisons to studies of other old, frail populations and the continuum of care model provide a basis for some assumptions regarding the characteristics of the RCF group. Such comparisons do not delineate the needs of this population clearly or adequately. Without adequate data, projections of demand cannot be undertaken, nor can the types of services needed by residents of these facilities be identified.

DEMAND FACTORS: THE CHANGING STRUCTURE OF HEALTH CARE

Numerous economic, social, and political factors now influence the state of long-term care and the search for community alternatives to institutional care. These include inflation, decentralization of health and welfare services (the New Federalism), fiscal crisis at the state and local levels, and the historical orientation of the medical profession toward acute care (Johnson & Grant, 1985). The following analysis looks at the realities of health care costs. It then examines the role of the federal and state governments in determining the demand and the supply of long-term care services.

Health Care Expenditures

The rising cost of health care services in the past decade has had a critical effect on public policy affecting older persons. The increases in health care costs are usually attributed to inflation, costly advances in medical technology, and demography, primarily the increase in the number of elderly consumers. While the elderly comprised only 11 percent of the population in 1980, they accounted for 29 percent of expenditures for personal health care. About half of all public spending for personal health care was for the aged (Fisher, 1980). The illnesses of the elderly tend to be long-term and chronic; they often require extensive and costly medical intervention, particularly in the final years of life.

Escalating costs in health care are evident in both the public and private sectors. Total health expenditures in the United States in 1985 reached $425 billion, an increase of 8.9 percent over 1984, and health spending amounted to 10.7 percent of the gross national product (Waldo et al., 1986). While 9 percent growth is clearly a significant increase, it is the smallest increase in health care expenditures in two decades.

Rising costs include the costs of both hospital care and long-term care services. Hospital costs reflect the slower rate of increase in health care expenditures cited above, with a growth rate of 6.1 percent in 1984; hospital expenditures, however, still accounted for 46 percent of all personal health care spending (Levit et al., 1985). More importantly, expenditures for long-term care continued to rise.

In 1984, $32 billion was spent for nursing home care, an increase of 8.9 percent from the previous year. Long-term care now amounts to about 8 percent of total health spending and to 9 percent of personal health care expenditures (Levit et al., 1985). In historical perspective, nursing home care "expenditures grew from $7.3 billion in 1973 to over 17.8 billion in 1979, an overall increase of 148 percent" (Johnson & Grant, 1985, p. 182); this figure had escalated to $24 billion by 1981 (Freeland & Schendler, 1983). While part of the growth in spending for nursing home care can be attributed to the use of intermediate care facilities for the mentally retarded (ICFMR), the aged population, which increased 2 percent in 1984, accounted for one-quarter of the growth in nursing home spending. Public financing of health care from 1965 to 1979 increased dramatically as a result of the Medicare and Medicaid programs and has since leveled off at about 40 percent of personal health care expenditures. In 1984 Medicare spent $63 billion (18 percent of total personal health care expenditures), and Medicaid, with federal and state shares combined, spent $37 billion (Levit et al., 1985). Public financing of nursing home care has declined since 1979, from 56 percent in that year to 49 percent in 1984, and it is obvious that a large part of the burden of financing care still falls on individuals and families.

Projections for health care spending in the coming decades cite a slow deceleration in expenditure growth, based on several trends. These include a moderation of overall economic inflation in the 1980s, restrained public spending, increased competition between providers in the health care industry, and the effects of cost-containment efforts implemented earlier in the decade. But the aging of the population and the new medical technologies may act as upward pressures on expenditure growth (Freeland & Schendler, 1983). Total public expenditures for health care are expected to reach $325 billion by 1990, with the federal government financing approximately 71 percent. Total costs for institutional care, including hospital and nursing homes, are expected to consume about 60 percent of personal health care spending (Freeland & Schendler, 1983).

To understand more fully the forces determining health care costs and projections for the future, we must comprehend the political and economic factors that currently affect spending for health and welfare services, including the major public health care financing programs. The way in which these programs have contributed to expenditures for health care and to current efforts to reduce these outlays can then be examined.

Fiscal Crisis and Decentralization

Fiscal crisis as a term has been widely used in the 1970s and 1980s to describe the fiscal problems faced by governments in the United States. Generally, the term "refers to the inability of government to meet current operating expenses, impending or actual fiscal deficits, defaults on government obligations, or other general fiscal problems of government" (Harrington et al., 1985, p. 115). O'Connor (1973) defined fiscal crisis as "a tendency for expenditures to rise faster than revenues" (p. 2), a tendency that may threaten the government's survival as a relatively autonomous entity. The same author referred to a "structural gap between the state expenditures and revenues" (p. 9), consisting of simultaneous tendencies toward an increase in demand for expenditures and a limit to the base of revenue.

The major focus of the fiscal crisis is the economic inability of state and local governments, in particular, to cope with a shrinking federal commitment to provide services. Several factors have contributed to the so-called crisis. These include declining tax bases, an inflationary and recessionary economy with rising interest rates, rising unemployment that increases demands on governmental support programs, and increased pressure from the federal government for states to pick up the costs of social programs while it simultaneously cuts the federal budget.

Typically, fiscal crisis may be treated in alternative ways. Governments can raise taxes to increase revenues. This step, however, can lead to taxpayer revolts that may further reduce revenues. Another tactic is to cut expenditures. Such cuts usually occur in services, in transfer payments, or in transfers to other levels of government.

The effects of state fiscal constraints typically hit hardest the areas of education, public welfare, and health. Since these areas consume more than half of all state public expenditures, they are major targets for reductions in future growth. Health care programs are particularly vulnerable. On average, health care now accounts for one-third of state human welfare outlays. During the 1960s and 1970s health care costs grew 40 percent faster than any other human welfare expenditures (Rogers, 1984).

The fiscal crisis prompted a closer look at the rising costs of health care cited previously. The federal government focused on reducing its share of support and on curbing the growth in health care. For the past two decades, however, planning for health and welfare services in general, and for services for the aging in particular, rested on the assumption of continued growth or at least maintenance of current levels of spending for health and welfare. Many of these programs, including the Older Americans Act programs, Medicaid, and Title XX social service programs, were designed to be administered by the states, but basic funding and overall policy decisions were made at the federal level. The fiscal crisis has played a critical role in efforts to curb health and welfare costs since 1978, especially challenging the assumptions of maintenance or growth. In particular, the cost containment strategies implemented by the federal government in health and social services have forced the states to deliver services with both declining federal support and declining state revenues. The primary state response to this dilemma has been to reduce overall services, through tightening eligibility requirements for programs, reducing service areas covered, reducing direct benefits, implementing utilization controls, and cutting personnel. The major impact of these reductions has been to limit services and benefits to the poor, through changes in Medicaid and the block grants for social services and special programs (Harrington et al., 1985).

The impact of the fiscal crisis has been exacerbated by what Estes et al. (1983) described as increasing decentralization of program and fiscal responsibility and increasing support for "the new Federalism" (p. 70). In the view of Estes, the philosophy of decentralization is part of recent conservative efforts to reduce federal responsibility for social needs. Thus, programs whose policies had been primarily the responsibility of the federal government have shifted more administrative, programmatic, and fiscal responsibility to the states (for example, Medicaid and Title XX Block Grants). In some cases local governments now have a larger role (for example, Older Americans Act programs). This policy shift has as its goal the lowering of the federal share of the health care budget. Changes in Medicare have reduced the federal contribution by increasing cost sharing by consumers, while changes in Medicaid programs have reduced the federal contribution by increasing the amount of costs that must be shared by the states.

The impact of the fiscal crisis and decentralization has resulted in multiple state efforts to redesign programs and reduce costs. Since the programs most affected by the federal cuts (Title XX and Medicaid) serve the most disadvantaged, the poor and the elderly are distinctly vulnerable: they are now dependent on benefits largely determined by state discretionary policies (Lee, 1980). The states vary greatly in their ability to absorb the fiscal and administrative responsibility for health and welfare programs. For example, those states hardest hit by the economic stresses of the last decade have been the least able to assume increased responsibility for support programs.

In addition, Chubb (1985) has argued that the policy priorities of the state, county, and municipal governments, which must now assume these responsibilities, differ from the priorities of the federal government. In particular, the lower levels of government must compete with one another for businesses and taxpayers. Therefore, they are less inclined than the national government to tax progressively or spend for social welfare. Others contend that the central government, with its larger constituency, presumably tends to serve broader and more diffuse interests. Smaller jurisdictions, by contrast, are seen as dominated by economic interests that allegedly exercise control to the exclusion of weaker, less organized groups. Minority rights are therefore more likely to be suppressed (Thompson, 1986).

In a variation on this argument, Estes (1979) maintained that decentralization leads to fragmentation of social programs. It transfers program responsibility to the state and local level, where the politicization of programs and priorities takes place among a more limited number of special interest groups. Thus, the extent to which a few special interests dominate the local political process shapes and creates greater variability in programs across state boundaries. Estes and Gerard (1983) have also contended that the states in general do not have the ability within their taxation limitations to generate the funds necessary to provide adequate social and health services to their residents.

On the basis of these beliefs regarding the states' capacity, some have argued that the changes in federal policy signal that "the federal government washes its hands of issues of equity and redistribution which, in our federal system, it alone can address effectively" (Brown, 1983a, p. 33). Serious questions can be raised about the states' fiscal capacity and the consistency of the states' commitment to equity in service delivery in a time of economic retrenchment (Thompson, 1986). Whatever the outcome of this shifting of responsibility in the coming years, it is clear that the states have made dramatic changes in an attempt to control health care costs. The pressure for residential alternatives and for deinstitutionalization of the aged is but one example. Thus, "In the search for alternatives . . . other forms of long-term care service are presumed to reduce the costs, thus benefiting state and federal governments" (Johnson & Grant, 1985, p. 185).

The cost containment strategies embodied in the recent changes in Medicare and Medicaid are particularly important to the growth and interest in alternative forms of care and to the overall changes in the health care sector. An examination of these changes and of the states' responses to federal policy illustrates the pressure for alternative forms of care.

Medicare and Hospital Cost Containment

Medicare, established in 1965 under title XVIII of the Social Security Act, was conceived as a federally operated health insurance program. It has been the principal source of public finance for acute care, mainly for the elderly. The program provides hospitalization and medical insurance for those persons over age 65 who are eligible for Social Security or railroad retirement benefits. In 1972, coverage was extended to include certain categories of disabled persons and to younger persons suffering from end-stage renal disease.

In recent years, policies designed to reduce public spending on medical care have targeted the increasing cost of Medicare. By 1981, Medicare's share of federal health spending amounted to $42.5 billion. Between 1974 and 1979, Medicare spending grew 150 percent. By 1985, Medicare spent $71 billion for health care, 19 percent of all personal health care expenditures (Waldo et al., 1986).

Only a small part of this growth can be attributed to increased enrollment, since expenditures per enrollee in the same time period more than doubled, accounting for 84 percent of total spending increases (Feder, 1983). Contributing to the increased costs per enrollee have been general economic inflation, increased utilization, and the reimbursement structure of the Medicare program, with its history of cost-based reimbursement. Projections made by the Congressional Budget Office predicted that Medicare spending would double again between 1982 and 1987 (Feder, 1983). As cited earlier, these costs have begun to show some slowing and stabilization, but control of costs is still a major focus for limiting federal spending in health care.

Hospital costs account for over 70 percent of Medicare expenditures (Feder, 1983). Hence, control of hospital and physician fees has been the target of major cost containment legislation in recent years. Two major approaches have been utilized within the Medicare program to reduce federal costs—increased cost sharing by beneficiaries through higher deductibles and copayments and the implementation of a prospective payment system for hospital services.

For the first time in the history of the program, major cuts were made in federal spending for Medicare in 1981 as a result of the Omnibus Reconciliation Act (OBRA). The cost to beneficiaries rose through higher deductibles and copayments. The policy of increased cost sharing has several rationales. First, it reduces federal costs for the program. Second, it aims to make consumers more aware of the real costs of care, thus motivating them to reduce unnecessary use. In addition, the high deductible mandated in the Hospital Insurance (HI) program supposedly encourages patients to utilize outpatient treatment instead of inpatient hospital care and to inhibit unnecessary or inappropriate use of skilled nursing facilities. In particular, it has been argued that the elderly, more often suffering from chronic conditions, could be better served in custodial situations rather than in skilled nursing facilities. This provision could result in an increased demand for residential facilities that provide some medical oversight.

Cost sharing may indeed reduce utilization and thereby reduce costs, but the impact of increasing copayments and deductibles is an acute hardship felt mostly by the poor or nearly poor elderly. Some have hypothesized that this hardship leads older people to postpone necessary treatment and forego the diagnostic testing necessary for lower-cost treatment in the early stages of disease. In such a scenario, questions of equity in service delivery are ignored, as they have been in debate on decentralization. Here, however, inequities occur not through state variation, but by the flat fee schedule used in the Medicare program. (Under the Medicare guidelines, physicians are paid a flat rate for visits. Since these reimbursements often do not keep up with market rates, the balance of the costs of physicians' visits must be paid by consumers.) The greatest economic burden falls on those least able to afford the costs of care.

While many older adults have felt the impact of increased cost sharing, the policy has had less overall impact on the use of nursing home care and community alternatives than have other federal changes. Specifically, dramatic changes in Medicare reimbursement have resulted from recent policy efforts focusing cost control on providers of care, that is, hospitals and physicians. These strategies have the potential to affect significantly the need for additional care settings for frail older people.

Perhaps the most important of these strategies was the introduction, through 1983 Social Security legislation, of the diagnostic-related group prospective payment system (DRGs). This system applies only to Medicare reimbursement in hospitals. Basically, the program provides for the classification of all patients into one of 468 diagnosis-related groups (DRGs), and the hospital receives a fixed payment per DRG to cover operating costs. These payments are calculated for each hospital as a function of area wages, rural or urban location, and number of full-time interns and residents on staff; in addition, capital costs and direct education are still included. The program was phased in over three years. By 1987 it was to be fully operational so that reimbursement to a given hospital for the operating costs of serving Medicare beneficiaries would be completely based on a national prospective payment system.

Essentially, DRGs limit both length of stay (LOS) for a given condition and also associated treatments that will be reimbursed. The incentive is for hospitals to discharge patients sooner and to provide only the most medically necessary services. If the hospital discharges the patient in less time than is paid for under DRG, the hospital keeps the difference as profit. If, however, the patient must stay longer than allowed under the DRG system, the hospital must absorb the additional costs of care incurred.

Some early evidence shows that the DRG system may have helped contain costs through earlier discharge. Length of stay declined from 9.3 days in 1983 to 6.7 days in 1984—the lowest level ever recorded (Levit et al., 1985). In addition, in the same period, overall admissions declined by 1.4 million (down 3.7 percent), and inpatient days were down 8.6 percent or 22.7 million (Levit et al., 1985). Some of this saving in costs may be offset by increased utilization of outpatient services and by the patient selection aspect of the DRG system. That is, only patients with a particular DRG may be admitted, primarily those who are less costly to treat. Other evidence, however, suggests the opposite trend. A recent report cites that "despite implementation of the prospective payment system, Medicare's share of the nation's hospital bill continues to rise, from 26 percent in 1981 to 29 percent in 1985. In 1985 alone, Medicare expenditures for hospital services rose 10.1 percent faster than the growth in all remaining non-Medicare hospital revenues, which increased 6.2 percent" (Waldo et al., 1986, p. 7).

Whatever the outcome in terms of cost containment, one of the most critical effects expected of the DRG system is the expectation of increasing demand for nursing home beds, rehabilitation sites, and home health services as patients are discharged earlier in the recuperative stages of their medical treatment. As Sorkin (1986) noted, "It is possible that patients receiving services in these settings will have more severe conditions and thus be more costly on the average than those treated before implementation of the DRG system" (p. 47). Thus, savings realized in the acute care setting may merely be shifted to other forms of medical and supportive care. Interviews with local providers support this hypothesis, with one nursing home administrator complaining that hospitals "now send me patients with open wounds!" (private interview, 1987). A recent study of the impact of DRGs on nursing homes in Portland, Oregon (Lyles, 1986) found that more than half of the respondents reported increased severity of illness among residents, shorter length of stay, increased prevalence of clinical problems, and increased use of medical supplies.

This increased demand for nursing home service comes at a time of documented shortages of nursing home beds in many areas, as a result of cost containment strategies in long-term care, for example, low reimbursement levels for Medicaid clients and tightening certificate-of-need requirements. The early discharge incentive, combined with changes in Medicare that cover more procedures that can be done at home, has also increased demand for home health services. A national survey of Area Agencies on Aging reported significant increases in the use of case management services and in-home skilled nursing following implementation of DRGs (Harlow & Wilson, 1985). Home health agencies have also reported an increase in sicker patients. They cite the need for specialized staff training in order to implement such procedures as intravenous feeding and hyperalimentary feeding (Harrington et al., 1985).

Preliminary evidence also suggests that the DRG system influences the long-term care system by reducing the number of hospital admissions from nursing homes and private home settings. Coe, Wilkinson, and Patterson (1986) reported significant age differences in such hospital admissions between their pre-DRG sample and the post-DRG sample, with the post sample significantly younger. They hypothesize that the older old are not being admitted unless they exhibit acute medical symptoms; as opposed to earlier years, they remain in nursing homes, private homes, or other alternative care settings that now provide higher levels of nursing intervention. The effects of the DRG system thus work to drive care out of the hospital setting and into other medical care settings.

In other words, the change might be pictured as "backing up" the system, with patients discharged from hospitals backed into progressively less care-intense settings as needed or as available. For example, a post-surgical elderly patient with skilled nursing needs is discharged to a nursing home as soon as the DRG limit is up. In order to keep as many beds available as possible for patients discharged from hospitals (patients often needing skilled nursing care), the nursing home will have fewer beds available for the less costly intermediate care patients. Nursing homes thus increasingly become responsible for the sickest and most costly patients. If, however, elderly individuals released from the hospital need intermediate level care, they may instead be sent home with intensive home health services. Another scenario is that these elderly people, with impairments that formerly would have required them to seek services in an intermediate care facility, will be placed in residential care or sheltered care alternatives. The potential, then, is that frail elderly people may seek out or be placed in care settings that are unsuited to their level of need. What was formerly considered a housing option has now become a medical care setting.

Hospitals, recognizing the potential income in providing these post-hospital services (and needing to compensate for the loss of bed utilization) have begun establishing relationships with or directly purchasing nursing homes. They thus insure the availability of skilled nursing beds when discharge is medically indicated under the DRG system. Some hospitals have also begun to plan skilled nursing units within their own facilities; these hospitals now own and operate their own home health care businesses. In fact, hospitals are moving into the home health business in increasing numbers. In 1984, 42 percent of hospitals nationwide offered home health services, and by 1985 this number was expected to increase to 65 percent (Glenn, 1985).

To summarize, these changes have a significant impact on the elderly and their ability to secure quality health care. In addition, cost containment strategies, such as prospective payment, may increase the demand for alternative forms of support and service delivery, such as home health and residential care alternatives. The impact of changes in the Medicaid program may have even more profound consequences for the expanding residential care industry, particularly as it serves the poor aged.

Medicaid: Cost Containment and the States

Medicaid, the combined federal and state program providing medical assistance to low-income persons, has been a particular focus of policy concern as expenditures have increased dramatically in the past decade. From 1978 to 1982, for example, total expenditures increased from $17.9 billion to $29.3 billion, representing an increase of 64 percent, while the consumer price index for the same period increased by 48 percent (Harrington et al., 1985). By 1983 this figure had increased to $35.6 billion and by 1984, to $37 billion (Levit et al., 1985; Sorkin, 1986). In some states, Medicaid is often the single largest program in the state's budget, accounting for about one-third of state and local health care budgets (Bovbjerg and Holahan, 1982). This growth has been attributed to several factors, including more intensive use of services, a broadening of additional services covered by Medicaid, and increases in prices (Holahan, 1983).

In particular, the rising costs of hospital and nursing home care, which in combination account for over 70 percent of Medicaid expenditures, have forced federal and state governments to enact cost containment measures to reduce outlays for medical care for the low-income and medically needy. At the same time, the fiscal crisis of the state has exerted increased pressure on the states to provide funds for social and medical care for the poor. Recent federal legislation, such as the Omnibus Reconciliation Act of 1981 (OBRA) and the Tax Equity and Fiscal Responsibility Act of 1982 (TEFRA), has only intensified this pressure by reducing the federal match for Medicaid assistance and allowing states to implement cost-sharing programs.

State responses to the legislative efforts of 1981 and 1982 have focused on changes in the variables that determine spending. These include eligibility, service coverage and utilization, provider payment, and other measures to reduce costs. Research shows that in response to the fiscal pressures of recent years most states have reduced eligibility and thus controlled costs, primarily by failing to index welfare standards to inflation (Bovbjerg & Holahan, 1982). Thus, as eligibles' incomes and assets have risen with inflation, more and more of these eligibles have dropped off the welfare rolls and lost Medicaid benefits.

In addition, states have dropped certain optional Medicaid eligibles, such as unemployed parents. The aged have fared better under utilization control mechanisms, primarily because many of the recipients are in institutions, and it is politically difficult to reduce coverage for such a vulnerable population. In addition, for many there is no feasible alternative to Medicaid support in a nursing home. For the noninstitutionalized elderly, cuts in Medicaid eligibility may only shift the costs of care to existing alternatives, such as private insurers or public hospitals and clinics. In either case, the state loses federal matching funds.

States have also made dramatic changes in methods of payment to providers, with the most critical efforts focused on hospitals. Since 1981 more and more states have opted to implement some form of prospective reimbursement for their Medicaid programs.[1] Since Medicaid provides for only about one-tenth of total hospital revenues, however, the incentive for hospitals to reduce costs as a result of the Medicaid prospective payment systems has been minimal. As cited above, reducing Medicaid reimbursement rates may only shift the costs of care to other providers or force cuts in beneficiaries.

Perhaps most critical to the discussion of care alternatives are recent Medicaid nursing home cost containment strategies. Nursing home expenditures have also been the target of cost containment measures because of the increasing share of total health costs expended for nursing home care. "Nursing home expenditures increased at a rate of 17.4 percent between 1980 and 1981 and 12.9 percent between 1981 and 1982" (Harrington et al., 1985, p. 125). Put another way, 43 percent of all Medicaid dollars were spent on nursing home services in 1983 (Sorkin, 1986).

States have made fewer changes in reimbursement for nursing home care than for hospitals following the OBRA and TEFRA legislation. The states have traditionally had much more control over nursing home costs, since they are the primary payer, with Medicaid providing about 49 percent of all nursing home revenues. The remainder is paid by private individuals. States have historically had greater flexibility in setting payments for nursing home care. By the 1970s, many states had already implemented restrictive nursing home payment systems in an effort to reduce costs. Any significant reductions beyond these previous efforts might seriously reduce the quality of care and affect the access of Medicaid recipients to care. Still, Feder (1983) pointed out that the 1981 federal legislative reductions may have "only marginally reinforced the already considerable fiscal pressure on states to limit their Medicaid spending," but the "result exacerbates a long standing shortage of nursing home beds for Medicaid patients, particularly those in need of costly care" (p. 48).

In response to OBRA, even greater flexibility was given to states by "softening reasonable-cost related reimbursement . . . so that now states are only required to pay rates that are reasonable and adequate to meet the necessary costs of efficiently and economically operated facilities" (Bovbjerg & Holahan, 1982, p. 47). In essence, states would now use the same standard of payment as that set for hospitals by the 1981 act. Recent research shows that states attempt to reduce costs mainly by implementing prospective payment systems for nursing homes. In addition, some states are participating in demonstration projects to provide long-term care services on a prepaid capitated basis; others are establishing community-based long-term care options through waiver programs for long-term care alternatives (Harrington et al., 1985).

In review, the changes in Medicare and Medicaid fiscal and programmatic options have had a definite impact on the elderly and the poor. The elderly, a primary consumer group of medical care, have faced increasing demands for copayments and higher deductibles, have encountered fewer choices in both the length and quality of hospital care, and, if poor, have suffered increasing restrictions on income and assets before attaining eligibility for hospital and long-term care assistance.

More Recent Federal Changes

Recent changes at the federal level will also have consequences for the levels of intermediate and skilled nursing facilities and for residential care facilities for the elderly. The Omnibus Budget Reconciliation Act of 1987 (U.S. Public Law 100–203, 1987) amended the Medicaid statutes by abolishing the distinction between ICF and SNF (except in the case of intermediate care facilities for the retarded), essentially combining them into one category of "nursing facility" by October 1, 1990. The amendments also upgraded staffing patterns by requiring that all ICFs and SNFs provide twenty-four-hour licensed practical nurse care seven days a week, with at least one registered nurse employed eight hours per day, seven days per week. Although it is too early to predict the overall impact of this change, a recent report on changes in the state of California predicted that: (1) those ICFs that cannot meet the more stringent fire and life safety regulations for an SNF will need a state waiver to operate as a nursing facility; and (2) some ICFs with substandard physical plants will have to be downgraded to a lower level of care (California Health and Welfare Agency, 1988).

These changes will certainly impact the demand for RCFs. In states where significant numbers of ICFs may be downgraded, these facilities provide a supply of existing structures for RCFs. In states where most nursing facilities are already licensed for SNF-level care, more RCFs may be needed to meet the needs of older persons who will no longer qualify for nursing care under the new regulations. How these statutory changes will affect the profile of nursing home and residential care residents can only be speculated about this time. The recent OBRA rulings however, are likely to have an impact similar to that of the cost containment measures described above (DRGs)—forcing the more frail populations into residential settings.

If, as outlined above, both Medicare and Medicaid shift service provision—and thus costs—to other levels of care, alternative care systems must be able to meet this demand. The alternatives in long-term care, both for types of service and reduced cost, have yet to keep pace with the growing need for service. While alternate care exists through families, home health agencies, foster care, and related residential facilities, the level of care available from these sources is limited. Further, use of these alternatives implies coordination of planning for elderly clients who will not be served under current cost containment strategies. Discharge planners must know and be able to assess the care needs of increasing numbers of critically dependent older people, but many of the care options are not designed to treat the intensity of service needs seen in these frail elderly. Monitoring quality of care in such a diverse array of health settings may also prove difficult. The lack of a consistent regulatory practice by states in monitoring home health care is an example of the lag between the demand for services and the quality assurance functions that must accompany new service provision. The same could be said for board and care facilities.

A review of the state's role in determining demand for nursing home care, and thus for alternatives, should provide a way to view these interrelated changes in the health care industry and set the stage for examining the supply aspects of long-term care.

SUMMARY: DEMAND FOR LONG-TERM CARE SERVICES

The focus of debate regarding the demand for nursing home and other long-term care services has centered on the availability of nursing home beds and on other alternatives to provide services in noninstitutional settings. The controversy over nursing home beds deals with whether demand exceeds supply and with the role the state has played in the process of limiting the availability of beds. Scanlon (1980b) argued that demand does exceed supply; Feder (1983) and Levit et al. (1985) cited the shortage of nursing home beds in their analysis of health care cost containment measures. Harrington and Swan (1985), however, noted that accurate occupancy rates are difficult to discern, so that any predictions regarding average occupancy and demand are suspect. The bulk of the literature, nonetheless, seems to support the belief that a shortage does exist and may be exacerbated by recent health care changes.

In a model defined by Paringer (1985), demand for long-term care service "depends, among other things, on the health status and the socioeconomic and demographic background of the individual, the price of the health service, the price and availability of substitute and complementary health services, the amount of resources available to the individual, and the individual's tastes and preferences" (p. 235). State discretionary policies in any one of these areas can alter demand.

For example, if states adjust eligibility requirements for nursing home care under Medicaid to include individuals with higher incomes, the change will, in effect, lower the price of nursing home care for those now included under Medicaid, thus increasing demand for nursing home services. Under an opposite adjustment, the states, by tightening eligibility requirements and implementing copayments or deductibles, can indirectly raise the price of long-term care and reduce the demand. A state's decision to offer optional coverage or expand alternative services, such as home health care under the Section 2176 (or the more recent Section 1915[d] of the Social Security Act) waiver program, may also reduce the demand for nursing home care while increasing the demand for substitute services to replace institutional care. Utilization controls, such as limits on weekend admissions and elective procedures, would similarly reduce the demand for hospital services.

Yet state action to reduce demand for one service typically increases demand for another. For example, if less restrictive Medicaid eligibility standards are implemented and demand for nursing home beds increases, an existing shortage of beds may shift the care of the elderly back on hospitals, where the elderly patient must wait until a bed is available. More recent evidence suggests that a nursing home bed shortage does exist, particularly for Medicaid patients. Nursing homes, unwilling to accept the lower reimbursement rates paid by Medicaid, increasingly deny access to those with low income, preferring to rely on private-pay patients. The Medicaid clients are either inappropriately held in acute care settings or else discharged to inappropriate care settings, such as foster homes or residential facilities, where health care follow-up is unavailable or inadequate. (Some monitoring of these discharges, at least for clients receiving state assistance, is now possible in Oregon; see Chapter 5.)

States, in response to the fiscal crisis and cutbacks in federal funding, have increasingly implemented policies to reduce utilization and costs of nursing home care by reducing demand. More stringent eligibility requirements, implementation of copayments, adoption of waiver programs for home health care, and experiments with prepaid, capitated systems of reimbursement are all designed to reduce demand for nursing home care. States have also implemented preadmission screening programs as a "gatekeeper" function (Scanlon, 1980). These programs determine nursing home utilization and serve as a tool for assessing the type of alternative care most suitable if nursing home care is not indicated. These systems reflect the belief that community alternatives are superior and that some individuals can be diverted from ever entering a nursing home if alternatives are available in the early stages of their impairment (Knowlton, Clauser, & Fatula, 1982). States have historically used, and recently tightened, certificate-of-need requirements and kept reimbursement rates low in order to limit or reduce demand for nursing home services (Weissert, 1984). By reducing profit through reimbursement, demand is also limited because potential investors are discouraged from entering the industry. (This policy may, however, work to limit both for-profit and nonprofit development.)

In particular, the use of community-based alternatives and lower levels of custodial care is one mechanism the states have chosen to reduce the demand for nursing home care. This policy has thus increased demand for these noninstitutional services. The questions remain whether enough of these services exist and whether quality of care can be retained to meet the needs of those elderly persons covered. Measuring the relationship between nursing home utilization and the availability and use of alternatives is difficult. The problem remains that the alternatives are rarely funded directly by Medicaid. Moreover, the alternatives do not exist in every locality. Scanlon (1980) found that nursing home utilization was related to the availability of personal care beds, with nursing home utilization declining in proportion to the personal care bed supply. Others (Dunlop, 1976) have found that utilization of home health services by Medicare recipients reduced the demand for nursing home beds. The recent federal changes described above will also affect the demand for nursing home beds.

Paringer (1985) summarized the changing market for long-term care services by emphasizing that

the net effect of a policy change in a particular market will depend on the ability of the market to respond to the change and the ability of other markets to provide substitute services. Increased hospital utilization is a likely response when there is a nursing home bed shortage and there are vacant beds in the hospital sector. If both markets are in shortage situations [as would be expected with recent hospital reimbursement changes under DRGs], it is more difficult for the hospital to respond to the increased demand for nursing home care. Under these circumstances, patients may need to seek other alternatives, perhaps including alternatives not traditionally considered part of the health care sector (e.g., board and care, congregate housing) to satisfy their demands for services. Additionally, some patients may go without care. (P. 246).

This discussion has emphasized the effects of public policy decisions, specifically recent cost containment strategies, on the demand for long-term care services to meet the needs of an increasingly frail elderly population. An analysis of current market supply should now provide additional information needed by policy makers in determining utilization, expenditures, and planning for long-term care services.

NOTE

1. In a prospective reimbursement scheme, "reimbursement rates are set in advance before services are rendered based on some formula of past expenditures" (Swan & Harrington, 1985, p. 138).

CHAPTER 3

Supply Factors in Long-Term Care and the Growth of Residential Alternatives

In an economic model the supply of a service is a function of the amount of the service that producers are willing to provide at the current market price. Hospital industry literature has shown that the factors that affect supply of long-term care services are similar to those that determine acute care services. That is, supply depends on four general factors: the basic structure of the industry (including average size, ownership, and concentration of firms); the costs of providing services (which are related to labor and construction costs); the technology available; and federal and state policy, including financing mechanisms (Paringer, 1985, p. 236).

These factors provide the framework for the following discussion of the residential care industry as it now exists. The data regarding residential care are scarce, but they provide at least a general picture of the type and amount of service provided. As in the chapter on demand, the importance of federal and state policy in determining supply will also be addressed.

STRUCTURE OF THE RESIDENTIAL CARE INDUSTRY

Any accurate discussion of the residential care industry is hampered by the multitude of housing and care alternatives encompassed in the term *residential care* (see Chapter 1). In fact, referring to the loosely organized array of foster homes, personal care homes, board and care homes, larger, almost institutional facilities, and others as an industry may be a misnomer. Nevertheless, policy and regulation have been directed at the full gamut of alternatives as if a true industry exists. The literature reflects the difficulty in defining the care options included under this rubric, a difficulty that leads to the wide variations in estimates of the number of facilities and residents. The literature does, however, provide a beginning for estimating the size and function of residential care.

An early 1954 estimate, based on a survey of thirteen states (Solon, Roberts, Kruger, & Baney, 1957), reported 2,627 domiciliary care homes with 33,243 beds and a population of whom almost 90 percent were 65 years of age or older. Projections from these data estimate that at that time approximately 9,000 to 10,000 homes with 90,000 to 100,000 residents existed (Sherwood & Seltzer, 1983). A nationwide survey completed in 1961 (Sherwood & Seltzer, 1983) reported 3,435 homes for the aged, 5,392 boarding homes for the aged, and 1,076 rest homes, for a total of 208,429 beds in these related, nonmedical facilities for the aged; it is not clear if facilities providing only room and board were included. These figures, if correct, imply a significant increase in residential care provision over a decade. While later statistics generated from studies conducted by the National Center for Health Statistics show a slower rate of growth, it is clear that, even before the advent of Medicaid, the residential care alternative was growing.

A later report by Booz-Allen and Hamilton Associates in 1975 cited 34,000 residential care facilities with a total of 270,000 beds (Mor et al., 1986). A 1982 report completed by the Office of the Inspector General (U.S. DHHS, 1982) estimated approximately 300,000 board and care homes in the United States, housing between 500,000 and 1.5 million residents. By contrast, Palmer (1983), using estimates based on a 1979 Government Accounting Office survey, reported about 600,000 residents of residential care facilities.

Many of these facilities serve the mentally disabled. Lakin et al. (1982) reported an estimated 90,000 mentally retarded persons in "private community-based" residences, while another national survey by Janicki, Mayeda, and Epple (1982) estimated that 49,000 mentally retarded adults resided in 6,300 facilities of this type. An earlier study by Sherwood and Seltzer (1981) using a figure somewhere between these two, estimated that between 60,000 and 80,000 mentally retarded adults resided in board and care homes in the United States; the majority of these resided in foster care facilities.

In addition, the Sherwood and Seltzer report (1981) estimated that, as of 1980, there were about 120,000 elderly domiciliary home residents in the United States; about 70,000 board and care homes existed in which one or more elderly persons resided. A recent nationwide survey by Reichstein and Bergofsky (1983) identified approximately 25,000 licensed and 5,000 unlicensed board and care facilities primarily for the aged. Another study estimated the board and care elderly population at approximately 285,000 (Teresi, Holmes, & Holmes, 1982). In recently published data collected from a national survey of state agencies that regulate residential care homes, Mor et al. (1985, 1986) estimated that in 1980 there were 29,282 homes serving 355,804 residents, with just under half of these residents aged 65 and over. A nationwide survey conducted by the Aging Health Policy Center estimated that 458,513 board and care beds in 1983 served a variety of dependent populations, including about 114,000 mentally disabled and 340,000 aged and physically disabled adults (Stone & Newcomer, 1986).

The wide discrepancy in the estimates may reflect not only demographic differences in the regions/facilities sampled but also state differences in policy and regulation, the ambiguity in definitions, differences in reporting systems across the states, nursing home reimbursement levels, and the level of State Supplemental Payment (SSP) to the SSI program. Indeed, there is wide variation across the states in the total number of licensed beds, and this variation is associated with state size (see Table 3.1).

Size and Facility Structure

In the most comprehensive study to date (Mor et al., 1986), the great variation in size and definition of residential care homes was verified. In their sample, residential care facilities ranged from 1 to 500 beds, with 37 percent having 6 or fewer beds, 27 percent having between 7 and 20 beds, and 36 percent having 21 or more beds. The median number of beds was 14. In another article, Sherwood, Morris, and Sherwood (1986) posited a convenient split for analysis between the small, "case-managed, foster-family-type domiciliary care living arrangements" and large, more medically oriented congregate housing. This split seems confirmed by the Mor et al. (1986) statistics. These differences in size and focus have been the subject of differences in regulation as well and will be examined further in the discussion of the impacts of state regulations on supply.

Mor et al. (1986) also found differences in the percentage of single rooms: 51 percent of the homes reported only one-fourth single rooms, 21 percent had one-fourth to one-half single rooms, and 28 percent had 50 to 100 percent single rooms. In addition, 47 percent cited fewer than three clients per bath, and approximately one-half reported the presence of heat-sensitive sprinkler systems. Many of these structural requirements may have been mandated by state regulations.

The variation in size and service capability of the facilities surveyed by existing research demonstrates the difficulty of assessing the field of residential care. Newcomer and Grant (1988) noted that, while nationally the small facilities (one to eight) account for two-thirds of the total number of facilities, the majority of RCF beds are in large facilities (fifty beds or more). Specifically, there may be acceptable variations between the very small foster home and the larger, more medically defined residential facility. Nonetheless, regulation of an industry with such wide variation in structural aspects is difficult. In particular, states face the challenge of establishing regulations that will allow both the small family operator and the large facility to afford the cost of necessary safety and structural requirements (for example, fire safety adaptations and kitchen facilities). When

Table 3.1
Number of Licensed Adult Residential Care Beds by Type of Facility, 1983

State	Residential Care [1]	Adult Foster Care [2]	Apartments [3]	Unclassified
AL	684	987	-	-
AK	325	16	25	226
AZ	3,641	0	1,369	0
AR	1,098	0	0	169
CA	91,853	0	0	0
CO	693	656	322	235
CT	4,390	441	109	0
DE	446	402	86	0
DC	-	-	-	2,518*
FL	38,092	3,643	16	0
GA	424	1,248	496	1,480
HI	3,956	0	0	0
ID	1,941	0	0	0
IL	133	0	0	9,084
IN	1,653	862	0	0
IA	17,565	100	0	100
KS	370	0	0	850
KY	8,227	1,388	0	149
LA	545	100	128	0
ME	3,294	732	0	0
MD	4,183	218	128	0
MA	8,856	99	2,096	2,607
MI	25,909	8,497	0	0
MN	3,222	0	0	1,686
MS	462	0	58	0

these requirements go beyond the ability of owners/operators to comply, supply will be affected.

Ownership

Descriptions of the ownership of residential facilities suffer from the lack of consensus on what constitutes residential care. If one includes publicly funded congregate housing, where some settings now offer additional supportive services, the overall industry picture changes. The only available statistics on ownership did not include congregate housing, however. The Mor et al. (1986) study found that 58 percent of the 156 state programs in their sample reported that all or most of their residential homes were family-owned and operated. An additional 15 percent of the states' programs reported that most homes were nonprofit organizations, such as those owned and operated by churches. In their sample only 19 percent of the programs reported having responsibility for the regulation and oversight of state or publicly owned facilities. In sum, "most programs have a mix of owner-operated and larger proprietary facilities under their jurisdiction"

Table 3.1 (*continued*)

State	Residential Care [1]	Adult Foster Care [2]	Apartments [3]	Unclassified
MO	12,417	314	90	0
MT	662	187	0	0
NE	3,366*	450	-	0
MV	815	94	0	0
NH	1,493	0	0	0
NJ	13,682*	40	438	1,878
NM	1,794	0	0	0
NY	33,225*	1,800	0	6,451
NC	14,589*	2,942*	8	0
ND	2,111	0	0	53
OH	3,150*	-	0	2,756
OK	2,102*	0	0	-
OR	3,687*	1,526*	231	0
PA	15,074	0	0	9,780
RI	300	63	312	0
SC	3,471*	0	28	0
SD	1,119	320	137*	0

SOURCE: Institute for Health & Aging (IHA). Unpublished Residential Care Facility Telephone survey. San Francisco, CA: IHA, University of California, 1984.

- Indicates data unavailable at time of survey.
* Indicates incomplete data.
[1] Residential Care Facilities include a broad array of settings (e.g., community care homes, personal care homes, domiciliary care homes, supervisory care homes, sheltered care homes, family homes, and group homes).
[2] Adult Foster Care refers to a specific program, usually licensed or certified by the state, which allows individuals to provide board and care services in their homes to a limited number of nonrelatives.
[3] Apartments refer to freestanding facilities in the community which include units licensed to provide board and care services.

(Mor et al., 1986, p. 408). In a second phase of the Mor et al. (1986) research, a survey of 230 residential care homes found 72 percent reporting ownership by a private person and 28 percent reporting ownership by a corporation.

The smaller, family-type foster care facilities are more likely to be family-owned and operated, while the larger, more institutional domiciliary and residential care facilities tend to be owned and operated by private corporations or nonprofit organizations such as churches or fraternal organizations. Unlike the current nursing home industry, residential facilities are still predominantly small and are owned and operated by families. The concentration of "firms" has thus remained minimal, unlike the trend in nursing home care, which has increasingly concentrated proprietary ownership in the hands of large, chain investors. Interestingly, this pattern of small, single-family proprietorship predominated in the early years of nursing home care. Changes in financing and regulatory policies favored the larger corporate facility, which could profit from construction incentives and economies of scale and make corporate chain ownership more profitable (Vladek, 1980).

COSTS OF PROVIDING SERVICE

Attention has been focused on residential care as an increasing proportion of the cost that has been paid by the federal government under SSI benefits and by the optional state SSI supplements. Thus, the very limited data available on the cost of residential care have centered on the rates allowed under the SSI program as administered by the states. SSI levels are set at the national level, and in 1987 maximum benefit levels were $340 for an individual and $510 for a couple. Moreover, in some states the state supplemental payment (SSP) is tied to specific definitions of licensed residential care facilities (Center for the Study of Social Policy, 1988).

Most state payments (inclusive of both SSI and SSP) are between $450 to $600 per month, but the level of SSP and types of living arrangements used to set payments vary by state. In 1987, 24 states provided state supplemental payments of over $150 per month for an adult with nonmedical long term care needs in a residential care facility. At least 16 states had SSP levels of $200 or more for the aged and other eligible groups. (Newcomer & Grant, 1988, p. 17)

In their 1980 national survey of programs regulating or monitoring residential care homes, Mor, Gutkin, and Sherwood (1985, p. 164) found "an average monthly client charge of $323." In states without SSI supplementation, this figure was approximately 33 percent lower, amounting to $216 per month. The survey also found that less than one-half of all residential care residents received SSI (43 percent), indicating that the majority of client payments came from private funds. Thus, if we assume that 350,000 residential care residents, "43 percent of whom are publicly supported, paid an average of $323 per month, nearly $600 million in public funds are devoted to supporting residential care homes" (Mor et al., 1985, p. 164).

These same authors noted, with the exception of their preliminary study, a total lack of information on the costs incurred by residential care home operators in providing service to their residents, despite the scope of public expenditures for residential care. In addition, no research has been located that describes the costs incurred in the larger, private residential facilities and private-pay foster homes. A review of rates and the author's experience in geriatric case management suggest that their monthly costs may approximate those of intermediate nursing care. (These rates may vary from $900 to $2,000 per month in the region reviewed.)

The Mor et al. (1985) research attempted to break the costs of residential care into cost components, including food, utilities, staffing, mortgage, and fees. On average, of the $330 monthly cost per resident, just over one-third was attributed to food, and just under one-third was attributed to staffing. Interestingly, the smaller homes exhibited higher proportionate food costs, while in larger homes the higher expenditures for staffing, utilities, mortgages, and fees were offset by lower food costs, perhaps obtained through economies of scale.

Of additional interest was the finding that aggregate resident characteristics were not related to staffing costs but were related to food costs. Staffing costs vary with facility measures (such as size and regulation) but not with the mix of residents served. Mor et al. (1985) have noted:

These findings run counter to the current emphasis on measures of case mix as predictors of costs in the nursing home industry.... It was expected that homes with "sicker" residents or residents that present management problems would have high staffing costs. Because such case mix measures were not related to differences in staffing costs, it is likely that home operators relied on other strategies to cope with the added resource requirements presented by those residents who were physically ill or difficult to manage. (P. 170)

This finding is of particular interest when examining the costs of higher-priced foster care and private residential care. While no hard data exist, both a review of recent marketing materials and experience in case management suggest that such facilities offer differential rate packages for residents requiring varying levels of care. While other cost factors in residential care, that is, food, mortgage and fees, and utilities, may remain stable or constant, it may be that only in the provision of direct resident care can profit margins be built. State regulations do, in some instances, set minimum staffing requirements, but these are seldom indexed to the case mix of residents. In other words, even if a larger portion of the resident population in a given facility needs more intensive assistance, the staffing patterns can remain the same. A facility may thus charge higher rates for these residents but maintain minimum staffing; in addition, they may save costs on residents requiring little or no additional care. Regarding the setting of rates, the rationale of higher staff cost for more intensive service may therefore represent an inaccurate picture of the real costs involved in providing care for the frail elderly in residential settings.

TECHNOLOGY AVAILABLE

The presence and cost of medical technology are less critical in long-term care than in acute, hospital-based care. In residential care, the technology of health care equipment may be much less significant than in acute, hospital-based care. Thus, for purposes of this analysis, a modification of Paringer's model (see beginning of Chapter 3) is needed. Using Webster's definition of technology as applied science, we will refer to technology here as the science of caregiving. It will refer to the availability, training, and skills of providers that affect the supply and quality of care. When training and licensing of providers are mandated by the states, these requirements also impact supply. In addition, applied science will refer to the actual services provided by these caregivers.

Personnel

Very little literature exists on staffing patterns or problems of operation and management in residential care. What does exist corroborates the split in residential care between small (fewer than six residents) foster-family situations and larger domiciliary, or congregate care settings. While both purport to provide room, board, and protective oversight to persons not needing medical care, the existing research reflects the large amount of medical care needed by this population. Although many state regulations provide explicit staffing requirements, such as staff-resident ratios, and anticipate management problems through regulations on emergencies, medication supervision, special diets, and security, there is wide variation by state, by size, and by purpose of facility. There exists, however, little self-report information on providers, their training, and their perceptions of operational problems.

The predominant staffing patterns in adult foster care include the "couple," often referred to as "mom and pop" homes, and the more prevalent pattern of a single female provider. In an early study of the Pennsylvania Domiciliary Project, Gutkin and Sherwood (1979) reported that over 50 percent of the providers were single females. Bradshaw et al. (1976) reported that 90 percent of providers in their Kentucky study were female. It has been hypothesized that widows living in their own homes constitute a potential supply of both facilities and personnel. The prevailing pattern also implies that most female providers are middle-aged to elderly (Sherwood & Seltzer, 1983). Similarly, in their survey of 230 residential homes, Mor et al. (1986) found that 78 percent of providers were female, with 48 percent of those providers between 40 and 59 years of age and 30 percent over 60 years of age. In addition, approximately 67 percent of providers had been in operation six years or more. By contrast, the larger homes, usually regulated under the auspices of the state department of health, were more likely to be "well-established, corporate . . . with paid staff and male administrators" (Mor et al., 1986, p. 415).

Existing research documents the need for training for providers in residential care. Serious management problems may arise when providers have inadequate training and experience to deal with the supervision of medications, incontinence, special diets, and behavioral problems (Newman & Sherman, 1977; Schneider, 1976; Roberts, 1974; Bradshaw et al., 1976). Newman and Sherman (1977) reported that 80 percent of providers surveyed in the New York state adult foster care study stated that they had no training whatsoever for providing care. These providers specifically cited the need for training in the psychology of aging. Providers in small "mom and pop" homes, in particular, have frequently been found to be unskilled in such fields as bookkeeping and records management and to be unable to interpret and thus implement the intricate state and local regulations affecting their operations (Dittmar & Smith, 1983). At the same time, Reichstein and Bergofsky (1983), in their analysis of state regulations governing RCFs, found that a "bare majority" required any type of staff training, with 24 percent requiring training for all staff and 27 percent requiring training for only some staff.

If this literature is representative and if the trend toward placing more frail individuals in community settings continues, the lack of provider training could significantly affect elderly residents of these facilities. Two outcomes are possible. The quality of care may be sacrificed as elderly residents with greater physical and mental impairments are placed in facilities where the goal, at least as formally stated, is to provide nonmedical care and supervision. Home health services may provide some of the medical supervision necessary for more physically frail individuals in community facilities, but few services exist for assisting providers with the mental health needs of residents or providing consultation on behavioral problems. Alternatively, the supply of residential facilities may be adversely affected. Providers may leave the industry because of the increased need for medical and management skills, if there is no concomitant increase in reimbursement or support from medical and social service programs.

On a more optimistic note, some states are now experimenting with training programs for foster care and domiciliary care providers in an effort to support and maintain existing providers. Many larger domiciliary or congregate facilities regulated by state departments of health already have mandated training and in-service requirements similar to those required for intermediate nursing facilities.

Once again, the lack of clarity regarding the role of community residential alternatives—housing or medical care—emerges in the paucity of training for residential care providers. If, as the regulations reflect, the facilities are nonmedical in nature, then the provision of medical services to residents who need more medical care becomes problematic. At present, these needs appear to be met, if at all, through a variety of means, including inadequately trained providers. If residential alternatives continue to provide care for a more frail population, these issues will have to be addressed.

Services Provided

Given the dearth of literature on RCFs, it is not surprising that little systematic information on the services provided has been found. One source of data concerning board and care homes providing personal care is the Master Facilities Inventory (MFI), compiled by the National Center for Health Statistics (NCHS).

These data are incomplete because the NCHS did not include domiciliary homes or boarding homes in its national survey. It did, however, provide some information on services provided in personal care homes or "rest homes," the larger, more institutional facilities, and some "extended care" facilities without nursing services. Services included in the National Health Survey of nursing and personal care homes include: help with dressing, shaving, care of hair; help with tub bath or shower; help with eating; rubs and massage; administration of medications or treatment; and special diet (Sherwood & Seltzer, 1983, p. 89). A U.S. Congressional Budget Office publication (1977) reported that in addition to personal care and room and board, some facilities defined by NCHS as board and care may include services such as laundry, recreation, and social services, with the latter rarely reported.

In their survey of state programs monitoring residential care homes of all sizes, Mor et al. (1986) found that certain services are mandated by varying state regulations. Of these services, medical access and medication supervision were almost uniformly required. Two-thirds of the programs required assistance with activities of daily living, including 60 percent of the programs that required help with personal care, but only 20 percent of the programs required facilities to provide rehabilitation services.

Little more is known specifically about services provided to aged clients in the smaller foster-home or family-care facility. While this type of facility has long been an option for the mentally impaired, only recently has it been often used to provide care for the elderly. Sherwood and Seltzer (1983) reported in their literature review that "the service emphasis in the foster care home tends to focus more on what can be considered 'informal' rather than 'formal' supports such as the creation of a 'homelike' atmosphere and integration of the resident into the family life of the provider" (p. 91).

In the study of the domiciliary care program in Pennsylvania, the most frequently provided services in the foster care homes included laundry (97 percent), personal shopping (83 percent), cleaning of environment (80 percent), and transportation to social activities (77 percent). In addition, 50 percent of providers assisted clients with their finances, and 65 percent supervised medications. In terms of personal care, 49 percent provided grooming, 37 percent provided bathing assistance, 26 percent provided dressing assistance, and 21 percent prepared special diets (Gutkin, 1980).

At least theoretically, residential care homes are nonmedical in nature, so it is somewhat surprising that the provision of medical services predominates. In their survey of 118 state programs monitoring facilities for the elderly, Reichstein and Bergofsky (1983) found that 82 percent required domiciliary care facilities to provide assistance with obtaining medical services, 81 percent required supervision of medications, and 42 percent required participating facilities to administer medications and treatments in accordance with physicians' orders. Given the lack of personnel training and the increasing mental and physical frailty of elderly individuals in residential care homes, the potential for poor quality care is great. More information is needed about the specific medical care needs of elderly residents of residential care homes and the ability of providers to insure that adequate care is given.

FEDERAL AND STATE POLICY

On the supply side, state discretionary policies influence the residential care market in much the same way that they affect the supply of nursing homes. In particular, the passage of regulatory policy and the levels and methods of reimbursement have a direct impact on the supply of residential facilities. For example, regulations that strengthen life safety practices, such as fire safety and physical plant requirements, usually increase costs, which may reduce investment incentives (Dunlop, 1979). Regulations that mandate staff-patient ratios, which increase wage costs for providers, may also act as a disincentive to investors.

The type (retrospective or cost-based, prospective by class, or prospective by facility) and level of reimbursement strongly affect facility profitability and thus supply. For example, reductions in Medicaid and SSI reimbursement act to reduce supply, while increases in Medicaid and SSI reimbursement may stimulate the market as new investors enter it and established providers expand or accept Medicaid clients. In their survey of state programs monitoring residential care homes, Mor et al. (1986) found that 56 percent of those responding "felt that low payment levels were the principal barrier to the entry of additional providers in the field" (p. 409). Stone and Newcomer (1986) noted that the current reimbursement method for board and care housing, based primarily on SSI benefit levels, is an "inadequate mechanism for encouraging the expansion of supply and upgrading of facilities to meet life safety and quality-of-care standards" (p. 205).

Supply, together with demand, obviously has important implications for access to appropriate care. In particular, if the supply of beds is limited and demand by private payers is high, access to care is especially problematic for low-income individuals who must depend on public subsidies that are not set high enough to compete with private payers. Stone and Newcomer (1986) noted that no study of residential care to date has analyzed how reimbursement levels affect supply and access on a national level. Their data from Washington state, where reimbursement rates were considered low in comparison to private market rates, did indicate low occupancy rates (less than one-third) by SSI-eligible persons in the available supervised housing beds.

It is also true that changes in federal reimbursement policy, changes that allow payment for alternative forms of care, also affect supply. This effect appears in the growth of community alternatives, including home health and residential alternatives, since the passage and implementation of Section 2176 of OBRA of 1981 and OBRA of 1987. These provisions granted DHHS the authority to waive existing Medicaid requirements to permit states to finance noninstitutional long-term care services. The way each state defines its SSI policies in relation to Medicaid policy changes, including income eligibility standards, supplemental levels, and the kinds of noninstitutional arrangements that can be supplemented, makes a significant impact on the demand for and supply of these residential services within the state.

In addition, federal or state programs that underwrite bond issues or provide loan guarantees also stimulate supply by reducing investment costs and fostering new construction. Government programs that offer low-cost loans for renovation of facilities also contribute to supply. One hypothesis is that programs favoring construction would benefit the larger, domiciliary, or congregate care facilities, while loans for renovation or improvements in physical plant and safety would benefit the smaller, family-type homes serving only a few individuals.

The number, stringency, and complexity of regulations impinging on RCFs can also act as a disincentive for providers. Stiff regulations were mentioned by 37 percent of program and policy makers in the Mor et al. (1986) survey as a problem for providers who wish to enter or stay in the field; 26 percent mentioned a lack of system coordination among agencies involved. Inspections are an example of these regulations; residential care homes are inspected for various purposes, including fire and safety, sanitation, food and health services, and compliance with resident rights and services as prescribed by state policies. In addition, some states use case managers to monitor the care of clients who are SSI recipients and reside in residential care homes. Facilities are thus subject to multiple agency inspections, an intrusion that may have a negative impact on the willingness of providers to continue operation within the regulatory environment. (No studies were identified that examined empirically the extent to which this "drop-out" phenomenon occurs or the factors or combination of factors that contribute most strongly to its occurrence.)

Mor et al. (1986) found that facilities monitored by state departments of health were significantly more likely to report having four or more inspectors than were homes regulated by other state agencies (which the authors refer to as "integrated homes"). Even in smaller homes, however, 32 percent reported having to respond to three or more inspection agencies.

Case management usually involves determining eligibility, placement, and referral to services and monitoring client status in the facility. While a minority of residential care clients receive this service, it is most likely to be required under regulations governing placement and reimbursement for SSI recipients. These clients more often reside in the smaller homes (Mor et al., 1985); providers see case managers' demands, as well as additional state agency regulations, as a major barrier to continued, profitable service provision. Mor et al. (1986) reported that, while policy makers see low reimbursement as the major disincentive, "regulatory demands are the biggest complaint of active providers" (p. 415). States are thus faced with the dilemma of implementing policies to upgrade the quality of these residential facilities without "regulating them out of operation" (Weeden, Newcomer, & Byerts, 1986, p. 185).

DISCUSSION: SUPPLY OF RESIDENTIAL CARE FACILITIES

This chapter has utilized an economic framework to examine the variables that affect supply of residential long-term care services, including the structure of the industry, the costs associated with providing the service, the technology available, and the impact of federal and state policy. While the literature is limited, it does reflect the crucial importance of existing income maintenance and health care policies in determining the quality and supply of alternatives. Since reimbursement and regulation are often the primary "creators" of a residential care picture, comparison of the development of residential care with that of the nursing home industry may provide some additional insight into the industry as it now exists and its future development.

Up until World War II, early nursing homes resembled many of the facilities now called residential care homes. In fact, most were small, housing fewer than ten residents, and were operated by the owner or his or her family. Many of these "mom and pop" facilities were run in existing family homes with minimal profit and no external financing. The years following the war, however, saw growth in the nursing home industry as GI loans were used to purchase new homes or expand existing ones for this purpose. The expansion of state old age assistance programs also increased the purchasing power of older persons in need of assistance. Still, external financing was limited.

In recent years, however, external sources have had a significant impact on the shape of long-term care, and several studies have provided empirical evidence to verify the factors that shaped the current nursing home industry (Dunlop, 1979; Pollak, 1979; Vladek, 1980; Scanlon, 1980b). These authors have confirmed, with little variation, that federal policies in the areas of income maintenance, health, and housing have influenced the marketplace more than any direct governmental decisions to encourage or discourage nursing home use. Thus, reliance on the large, more institutional nursing home for care may have been an unanticipated consequence of other social legislation.

The past thirty years have witnessed a number of specific legislative decisions that contributed to the growth of nursing home use. These include the passage and subsequent direction of Medicare and Medicaid, Supplemental Security Income, emphasis on deinstitutionalization of the mentally impaired, and the structure of these systems, which limited reimbursement for nonnursing home alternatives. These factors, combined with increasing numbers of older people with greater purchasing power, fueled the demand for nursing home beds. Other variables were simultaneously at work both to encourage the growth of facilities and, more recently, to limit supply.

The nursing home industry began a major growth period with the availability of funds provided through the Hill-Burton Act of 1946. Hill-Burton funds for the construction of public and voluntary nonprofit nursing homes became available after 1954. The real boom, however, did not begin until legislation in 1956 that authorized the Small Business Administration (SBA) to make loans to proprietary nursing homes. In 1959, the availability of Federal Housing Administration mortgage insurance for newly constructed facilities further promoted the growth of the industry. Medicare and Medicaid reimbursement under the reasonable cost formula in 1965 provided additional financial incentives for increased nursing homes beds. The more recent growth of investor-owned chains, market speculation, the formation of a private bond market for nursing home development, and the expansion of leasing and merging contracts to improve economies of scale in chain operations have all contributed to the supply of nursing home beds (Lane, 1981; Harrington & Swan, 1985).

At the same time, constraints on nursing home growth have also been at work. The imposition of regulatory controls has had a primary constraining effect. These controls largely followed the passage of Medicare and Medicaid in 1965. The physical plant requirements mandated for Medicare and Medicaid participation acted as a constraint on facilities, particularly the small homes. In addition, the development of more stringent standards for patient care and for monitoring patient abuse, following congressional nursing home investigations, have made entrance into the industry more difficult. The 1972 amendments to Social Security mandating fire safety constraints limited the entry of new investors and forced substandard facilities out of operation. The Medicare and Medicaid Fraud and Abuse Amendments of 1977 further restricted the profit incentive in poor patient care.

A key factor inhibiting the growth and profit potential of nursing homes was the enactment of the National Health Planning and Health Resources Act of 1974, which mandated Certificate of Need (CON) requirements. While the original legislation was directed toward the control of hospital bed supply and occupancy rates, many analysts agree that the certificate-of-need process has had a much more substantial impact on nursing homes than on hospitals (Vladek, 1980). In addition to limitation of the overall supply of nursing home beds, others note that the CON franchise has been used strategically in some states to attract private-pay patients while restricting the number of public-pay individuals served (Lane, 1981).

At present, most analysts agree that demand (increasing numbers of frail older individuals and the lack of appropriate alternatives) has fostered capital investment in nursing homes. These same analysts assert that the current regulatory environment has contributed to a lag in the supply to meet this demand. The present nursing home marketplace is seen as one of excess demand, with particularly difficult issues of access for Medicaid recipients. As Lane (1981) noted, "As long as the public pay rate falls below the actual cost of services to an individual, there is no economic incentive to expand the market" (p. 32).

What are the differences and similarities between the nursing home market and the residential care industry? Residential alternatives are still in the developing stages. The majority of providers are still small-scale operators, functioning primarily in private homes housing six or fewer clients. Few government incentives, certainly none on the scale of the Hill-Burton and SBA legislation, promote growth of residential facilities. What does exist, primarily through the state SSI programs, Section 2176 (and now, Section 1915 [d] and [c]) programs, and Title XX, provides only modest support for those facilities serving the low-income. With current payment levels, little incentive exists for providers to remain in service or to enter the field. Supply is not limited at this time by the certificate-of-need process, except in states where CON requirements do apply to large domiciliary or congregate facilities and/or those residential facilities attached to larger nursing home arrangements.

It is especially true that until passage of the Keys Amendment, which encouraged states to develop regulations for residential facilities, few government-directed regulatory barriers existed to market entry. As states have implemented more stringent regulations in response to the Keys Amendment, more providers are faced with physical plant, staffing, and patient care requirements that may be difficult to meet. As with the development of the nursing home industry, these requirements fall most heavily on the small operator. As Vladek (1980) noted, "As regulatory activity increases, smaller firms tend to consolidate, sell out, or drop out, and that has clearly been the case with nursing homes" (p. 168). While most state regulations concerning residential homes discriminate between large and small facilities, with fewer requirements for smaller, family-type homes (Sherwood & Gruenberg, 1977; Reichstein & Bergofsky, 1983), regulatory demands are still a powerful disincentive to providers (Mor et al., 1986). The alternative side of the size factor is that the plethora of small, less regulated facilities makes it much more difficult to implement quality control and contributes to the current lack of knowledge regarding the costs, extent of services provided, and resident characteristics.

The impact of federal and state governments on residential care is also minimized by the lack of direct funding for this form of care. Functioning outside the traditional mechanisms of direct Medicaid/Medicare funding, the ability of the government to fuel growth through reimbursement or restrict growth by withholding reimbursement is limited. The impact of this structure is yet to be measured in the field of residential alternatives. Yet there is a growth in demand. With this increase, particularly for private clients, interest in assisted living has been shown by many of the same developers and investors found in the retirement industry. The private consumer is still the primary buyer of residential care services. Both developers and consumers have incomplete knowledge of the product. Residential care is a relatively new commodity, with great variability in the size and type of service offered. It is, on the whole, a smaller, less visible market.

The market for residential care both resembles and differs from that of nursing homes or retirement facilities. Some of these variations in market structure are

Figure 3.1
Variability in Market Structure: Nursing Homes and Residential Care

Nursing Homes	Residential Care
Certificate of Need (CON) required – barrier to market entry, limits supply	Limited CON certification
History of economic incentives for facility growth – Hill-Burton Act – SBA loan legislation – FHA mortgage insurance – Private bond market	Few economic incentives for facility growth – Limited state bond issues
Government primary buyer of services (State & Federal government provide 57% of receipts) – Incentive for growth	Private consumer primary buyer of services
Number of consumers known to some extent	Number of consumers unknown
Less variability in services provided	Greater variability in services provided
Larger, more visible	Smaller, less visible, less consumer knowledge of product
Greater government involvement in regulation/quality control	Less government regulation, more difficult to implement quality control measures
Profitability less than in past, but still viable	Little known about costs and profitability

reviewed in Figure 3.1. While the development of RCFs and nursing homes has proceeded on a similar path, the level of government intervention has been quite different. The futures of both industries are intertwined, especially in light of recent cost containment strategies implemented in the hospital and nursing home sectors. The effect of regulations and reimbursement will play an important role in defining the future of residential care, as will more knowledge of the consumers of these community alternatives. The challenge is to strike a balance between insuring quality care through regulation, reimbursement, and other strategies and not forcing low-cost, less restrictive alternatives to leave the market because of an excess of regulatory intervention.

Whether the future of RCFs resembles the history of nursing homes is a question that remains to be answered. No government has directly intervened to fund the expansion of such facilities, but the development of regulation proceeds slowly. The following chapters examine in more detail the development of regulations. This analysis will provide an additional framework for discussing the role of residential care and its ability to meet the demand for services. It should also allow speculation on the resemblance between the historical development of nursing home care and the future of residential care.

CHAPTER 4

Development of a Policy Issue and Regulatory Response

To examine policy developments in a given social problem area, one must first understand the factors that give rise to an "issue." Bardach and Kagan (1982) point out:

> The growth of regulation is not merely a product of the steady and relentless forces of logic and political and economic interests. Regulatory victories, as well as initiatives, are products of intermittent events or "occasions" that fire political imagination.... Most prominent are physical catastrophes; scandals that expose presumptive laxity, corruption, or incompetency in the regulatory agency; dramatic scientific discoveries; flare-ups of racial or intercommunal violence; and changes in administration. (P. 22)

Catastrophes most commonly initiate action. Nowhere is this process more evident than in the regulation of care for older people. In the past two decades, the nursing home industry has been the target of seemingly endless investigations of abuse and neglect. Beginning with in-depth newspaper investigations, followed by Senate and House special hearings that culminated in massive federal reports (U.S. Congress, 1974), and numerous volumes describing the underside of care (Mendelson, 1974; Moss & Halamandaris, 1977; Vladek, 1980), documentation of the excesses of treatment or the lack thereof has been substantial. In response to this evidence, public policy on services to the elderly has been legislated through the Social Security Act and the Older Americans Act. Federal and state governments have implemented layer upon layer of regulatory statutes, primarily linked to reimbursement through Medicare and Medicaid. Public awareness and policy responses in other care settings, such as board and care or RCFs, appear to be following a similar pattern.

Board and care facilities have existed for many years, primarily to provide food, shelter, and minimal protection for the chronically impaired, the dependent elderly, the mentally dysfunctional, and the disabled. In the past decade, a combination of factors, including the deinstitutionalization of mental patients, the growing fiscal constraints on state and local governments, the rising costs of health care and subsequent cost containment efforts, and the focus on community-based alternatives to costly nursing home care has increased the use of and interest in board and care and other residential alternatives. The use of "less-institutional" environments has been seen as a means to reduce the high costs of institutional care and to promote greater independence and life satisfaction (Harmon, 1982). As Kane and Kane (1980) have tersely noted, "Alternatives are pursued in hopes that they will be better and cheaper" (p. 250).

While board and care and other residential alternatives may be viewed as potentially valuable resources in the long-term care continuum, the lack of consensus regarding their identity and nature has been problematic. As described above, many are small, housed in private dwellings that may not meet adequate safety standards, and managed by individuals with few administrative skills or substantive knowledge regarding the social, psychological, or health needs of aged and disabled persons (Mor et al., 1986).

Problems in these facilities have recently been highlighted after a rash of boarding home fires and exposure of substandard conditions received national attention (U.S. GAO, 1979). Solomon (1982) stated that "reports of financial mis-dealings, deprivation of civil rights, physical abuse and neglect, deaths and injuries caused by preventable fires, starvation, and mismanagement of medications have emerged over and over again during the last ten years" (p. 2). In particular, the deinstitutionalization of mental patients into less costly community board and care homes has focused attention on the inadequacies and lack of governmental oversight in the growing industry of residential care.

Perhaps most important to understanding the federal response to regulating the board and care industry is the private nature of these institutions. While some board and care homes are in private residences, others are in hotels converted to care sites; still others are new, expensive buildings designed especially for this purpose. Unlike nursing homes, which receive funds from Medicare and primarily Medicaid, residential care facilities receive no direct federal reimbursement for supervision and/or care. Indeed, state policy makers have no clear understanding of the role of residential alternatives. For example, do they offer merely shelter and supervision, or do they provide care? Specifically, to what extent is medical care provided? For the most part, board and care homes are privately owned, for-profit institutions. The states, however, have increasingly placed low-income mentally disabled, physically disabled, and frail aged persons directly into these facilities, to relieve the high cost of institutional care, again with the goal of "normalizing" residents. Supplemental Security Income (SSI) checks have thereby become one of the main sources of payment to board and care homes. Although some states augment these payments with state funds, most SSI payments are underwritten by the federal government.

Before discussing the policy response to the inadequacies apparent in many residential facilities, we need a framework for analyzing this response. Three "lenses" provide a means for analyzing both the broad policy initiative at the federal level and the implementation that occurs within the federal and state governments. These include the organizational environment in which policies arise, the nature of implementation of policy, and the historical influences in the development of regulation for housing and care of the elderly.

FRAMEWORKS FOR POLICY ANALYSIS

Organizational Process Paradigm

Graham Allison (1971), with his examination of the United States role in the Cuban missile crisis of 1962, offered a particularly useful framework for policy discussion in the organizational process model. In his analysis, the governmental process model is an alternative framework to the more traditional "rational actor paradigm" in which government action is portrayed as "action chosen by a unitary, rational decisionmaker, centrally controlled, completely informed, and value maximizing" (p. 67). In his conceptual model, on the contrary, government behavior can be viewed "less as deliberate choices and more as 'outputs' of large organizations functioning according to standard patterns of behavior" (p. 67). A condensed summary of his model will here suffice to provide a framework for analyzing the federal response to the problems identified in board and care facilities.

First, Allison defined the basic unit of analysis as organizational output. Governmental action manifests itself in organizational outputs, limited in range by organizational history. "Existing organizational routines for employing present physical capabilities constitute the range of effective choice open to government leaders confronted with any problem" (p. 78).

The organizing concepts of the model include: a large cast of actors functioning as an organization; a factored approach to a given problem in which various aspects may be parceled out to numerous organizations, each with its own sphere of power and influence; a tendency to "parochial priorities and perceptions," because of the narrow aspect of the problem to which each organization must address itself; and the overriding propensity to approach problems as reenactments of preestablished routines (p. 81). In generating output, the activity of organizations takes place in the following steps.

1. The goals of the organization arise as a result of constraints defining acceptable performance. The constraints originate from relationships with other organizations within the government, special interest groups and influential cit-

izens, statutory authority of the organization, and dynamics of power within the organization itself.

2. There is "sequential attention to goals" (p. 82). Organizations perform their functions based on procedures designed to facilitate understanding across the subunits within the organization. These "standard operating procedures (SOPs)" allow individuals to perform tasks with minimal cues but often render organizational behavior "unduly formalized, sluggish, and in particular instances, inappropriate" (p. 83). These SOPs cluster into "programs and repertoires" (p. 83) that determine organizational behavior. The number of programs and repertoires is usually quite limited and cannot be changed for individual or unique circumstances.

3. Organizations generally avoid uncertainty by negotiating relationships with other government organizations in the areas of budget, responsibility, and established practices. When scenarios designed in advance to reduce uncertainty cannot be called upon to address a problem, the organization engages in "search," with the search constrained by established routines, biases of given actors with specialized training, and even communication within the organization.

4. Organizational learning and change do occur, although usually slowly and incrementally as new situations and responses evolve and become incorporated in existing routines and practices. In a few cases, however, marked changes may be possible:

    a. A budget feast occurs, and organizations begin to implement program changes that have been waiting for fiscal increase.

    b. Prolonged budgetary famine may force major cutbacks in previously well-established programs.

    c. Dramatic performance failures, often apparent in major catastrophes, may force change because of pressure on the organization from outside authorities.

Finally, it is important to review this conceptual model's approach to organizational options and their administrative feasibility. Allison postulated that the number of alternatives open to a given organization is limited in number and character. The potential alternatives differ from those that might be put forth by experts or by the public consumer, based on the following several characteristics of organizations.

1. "Alternatives built into existing organizational goals [for example, cost containment strategies translated into regulation of an industry to provide less costly care than federally funded nursing home care] will be more favorably reviewed." In contrast, "review of alternatives contrary to existing organizational goals [for example, providing greater reimbursement for board and care facilities through federal programs] will be poor" (p. 90). These proposals will probably encounter resistance. Concurrently, projects or programs that demand that units of the organization depart from established programs "are rarely accomplished as designed." (pp. 93–94).

2. "Alternatives requiring coordination of several organizations [for example, DHHS, Department of Housing and Urban Development, Administration on Aging, Health Care Financing Administration, older American advocacy/oversight groups] are likely to be poor" (p. 90). Again, accomplishment of programs designed under these constraints is rare.

3. "Alternatives in areas between organizations [for example, housing design for both public and private facilities] are likely to be poor" (p. 90).

Allison's model is particularly useful for examining the way in which DHHS, functioning within the constraints outlined, developed its guidelines for the Keys Amendment and subsequent revisions in an attempt to provide oversight for the residential care industry. More about the applicability of this model will follow the delineation of two additional frameworks.

Implementation: A Theoretical Perspective

While the development of policy may frame the programs designed to bring about reform, the implementation of policy often determines actual change. In his theoretical perspective, Martin Rein (1983, p. 113) described the translation of policy into practice as "the politics of implementation." Rein set out a framework, based on three imperatives—the legal, the bureaucratic, and the consensual—to examine implementation as a process in which conflicts among the three are somehow resolved. A summary of the three will clarify his perspective.

First, the legal imperative implies that actors in the implementation process must do what is legally required by the legislative mandate. In some instances, this imperative for legal compliance will be stringent, depending on the prestige of the committee in which the bill originated, the expertise of the members of the committee, the degree to which disagreements regarding the mandate were worked out before passage, and overall support for the law by legislators and the public. Rein (1983) postulated that "when these factors reinforce each other, the legal imperative will be most strict during implementation" (p. 120). By contrast, the legal imperative may be less powerful when legislative mandates are left intentionally vague. This situation has often been the case with domestic social programs. It occurs more often when swift passage of the legislation is necessary, when there is little apparent national understanding of and consensus regarding concrete methods for implementation, and when alternative policies are controversial, making it politically risky to outline a clear and unambiguous policy choice.

Second, the rational-bureaucratic imperative indicates that "the law still will be put into effect only if it does not violate the civil servants' sense of what is reasonable or just" (Rein, 1983, p. 120). Several bureaucratic perspectives are incorporated under this imperative, including "consistency of principles" inherent within the law itself, "workability" of the program created (or what professionals and managers see as feasible), and a concern for "institutional maintenance, protection, and growth" (Rein, 1983, pp. 121–122).

Third, the consensual imperative suggests that the interest groups affected by the mandate are usually paramount in the implementation process, to the extent of subordinating the legal and bureaucratic imperatives. This result usually occurs when a governmental agency is new or weak or under pressure from within and without or when an agency has been brought into existence by pressure from interest groups that have a strong hold on legislation affecting programs implemented by the agency. As Rein (1983) noted, a shift in power among the interest groups involved will signal a parallel shift in the implementation process.

Rein also outlined discrete stages of implementation, including guideline development, resource distribution, and oversight. He posited that each of the imperatives operates at each stage of the process. It is important to this analysis that Rein gave great emphasis to the development of guidelines. As he noted, it is an enormous challenge to draft administrative guidelines that both adequately reflect the intent of the legislation and are reasonable to managers. Decisions at this stage include whether to express merely a desired result or outline in detail the specific requirements for achieving the result and whether the mandate should require retroactive or proactive compliance. The discussion to follow regarding the drafting of federal regulations to implement the Keys Amendment and the subsequent regulations developed by the state of Oregon will validate Rein's emphasis on this stage of development.

The second stage of implementation includes the authorization-appropriation-disbursement strategy of funding, which can severely affect the implementation process by delays in any or all phases.

The third and final stage, oversight, involves "monitoring, auditing, and evaluating" (p. 127). Rein viewed monitoring as the least publicized but oft-used mechanism not only to review implementation, but to revise policy throughout the process by use of circulars and memos redefining goals and regulations. Confusion regarding the channels for reporting of compliance is common. Monitoring functions may change over time as subsequent revisions of the legislation become law or as agency roles and functions are redefined. In optimal conditions, the outcome of the oversight process should be that the various forms, including monitoring, auditing, and evaluation, act in a circular manner "altering legislative intent and administrative practice" (Rein, 1983, p. 129).

Rein then outlined environmental conditions that can critically influence implementation. In this analysis of the implementation of policy to regulate residential care, these conditions take on particular importance. The first condition, goals saliency, implies that "policies differ in how clearly they state what aims should be accomplished, whether these aims should be accomplished immediately, and whether they are more symbolic or more realistic" (Rein, 1983, p. 131). When the goals of new programs are unclear and when there is little precedent to provide guidance, weak and general guidelines often emerge. When there is confusion or lack of knowledge regarding details of actual implementation, there is seldom a mandate to accomplish within a specific time frame. Subsequently, some policies become more symbolic attempts to address issues that are politically difficult, unclear, or unfeasible given current funding and level of political/community support.

The complexity of the implementation process is also important. In Rein's (1983) view, "Implementation is also a function of the number of levels, the number of agencies, and the number of participants who have a say in the process or are able to veto any stage along the way" (p. 132). Two points of view have developed regarding the participation implied in this process. The first posits that high levels of participation constrain decision making. Such participation can make it more difficult to reach consensus and may make it difficult to focus on the original priorities of the mandate. The opposing view stresses that complexity itself provides protection from rapidly implementing policies that may have been hastily developed without adequate levels of participation during the legislative process.

Finally, "implementation is also a function of the type and level of resources required for action. . . . Not all legislation requires that resources take the shape of a direct outlay of expenditures" (Rein, 1983, p. 133). In more and more instances, federal policies and guidelines may require (as in the case of the Keys Amendment) that the outlay originate with the implementing bodies, in this case the states. Rein distinguished between legislation "designed to regulate the standards of products or the performance of individuals, firms, or agencies" and legislation that provides "incentives or distributes public largesse in the form of services or cash" (p. 134). When looking at implementation among agencies that serve different functions, such as administering programs, dispensing funds, or regulating behavior, Kaufman (1973) found that administrative feedback varied by agency function. One would assume that implementation would be carried out to differing degrees under different sets of political and administrative constraints. Regardless of function, adequate resources are crucial to the effective administration of program mandates.

Rein's framework implies a process of implementation in which opportunities for altering the intent of the original mandate occur at all levels of practice and in which constant pressure to achieve a consensus among all actors in the implementation process is present. Rein thus concluded that "in general, clear, salient, and realistic goals that can be implemented simply and that are supported by adequate, but not plentiful resources will lead to programs in which there is minimum discretion, little deviation from the policymaker's intent, and maximum consensus among implementators" (p. 135).

The two models described provide a useful framework for tracing the passage of the federal legislation aimed at residential care and for examining its subsequent implementation and revisions. In addition, I would argue not only that the organizational history and existing organizational routine constrain the choices open to policy makers, but also that the history of regulation in long-term care (based on the philosophical approach to social welfare in the United States) has limited the range of options open to consideration by government leaders. Contemporary theories of federalism and constitutional issues also constrain policy makers and define the role of federal and state governments in the implementation of policy.

Historical Influences

Residential care, like other forms of care provision for the dependent, has developed in an incremental manner in response to changing social forces rather than in a deliberate and comprehensive fashion. Legislative and financial organizations have often developed after the development of care options in order to regulate existing modes of operation, with the aim of improving these often fledgling efforts. The following discussion provides a brief history of the development of nursing homes and residential care and examines a few of the factors that have influenced the character of regulatory policy in these industries.

Modern nursing homes and residential care facilities can trace their history through three primary modes of care. These include the almshouse or poor farm, which had been the primary mode of care for the indigent and aged throughout the nineteenth century. The second was the private home for the aged, which developed around the turn of the century. First established by charitable organizations, these homes were designed to care for the healthier elderly who had limited income or no family. The third has been the proprietary boarding home, which also emerged around the beginning of this century but focused its efforts on those older persons able to pay for their care. As the residents aged, many facilities had to add nursing staff and thus gradually evolved into nursing homes or care homes with infirmaries. All these forms of care were considered the responsibility of local governments and were not regulated with any consistency, if at all.

Federal involvement in social welfare, as well as the growth of the nursing home and board and care home, however, can be traced to the Great Depression and to passage of the Social Security Act of 1935. Specifically, Title I of the act established a federal program of Old Age Assistance (OAA) in the form of grants-in-aid to states; this was a noncontributory, means-tested old age pension. One condition of the federal grant system forbade OAA benefits to individuals residing in institutions. This restriction reflected the philosophical acceptance of a cash grant benefit that would allow individuals to remain in the community. Individuals' control of benefits was also seen as a way to reduce the stigma attached to welfare programs. In addition, the federal restrictions on grants to states provided a ceiling on the federal contribution (which states were to match up to certain amounts) but provided no minimum contribution. States were thus free to supplement the federal expenditure with as little, or as much, as they desired. Eligibility guidelines were left to the states, with only minimal federal requirements imposed.

The OAA provisions greatly expanded the numbers of elderly persons able to purchase boarding home or nursing home care or to be maintained in their homes. Thus, for many older persons, Social Security now allowed them to remain at home until they needed nursing care. This change fostered the transformation of many boarding homes into nursing homes. During the decades 1940–60, the proportion of institutionalized elderly residing in "group quarters" declined from 41 percent to 12 percent, while the proportion residing in nursing homes increased from 34 to 72 percent (Dunlop, 1979). Nevertheless, these facilities had numerous problems because, although more funding was now available, few if any standards existed for their operation (Baggett, 1983).

As the demand for nursing homes increased, many of the existing residential facilities found it necessary to add nursing care and other medical services. In a spiraling cycle, additional staff members were required to increase the number of clients who could be served, while more clients were required to provide financial incentives for providing more intensive and costly care. Some facilities, having no experience in providing this scope of medical assistance, became overcrowded and unsanitary. The potential for abuse grew.

Additional legislation, particularly the 1950 amendments to the Social Security Act, nurtured the development of health care in these facilities, many of which began to resemble the larger institutions we now call nursing homes. Taking into account the shortage of available beds and the growing dissatisfaction with proprietary care, the first provision of the amendments lifted the prohibition of payments to residents of public medical facilities. The second provision allowed, for the first time, direct payments by public welfare agencies to the actual providers of health services, rather than to the beneficiaries (the first limited support for vendor payments so critical to the Medicare/Medicaid programs). This legislation also required that states establish a system for the licensing of nursing homes, but the requirements were minimal, great variation existed by state, and no provisions were made for enforcement (Vladek, 1980, pp. 40–41).

Since the early 1960s, nursing homes have developed as *the* specialized settings for delivery of long-term care for the elderly. Few questioned the medical model employed for their development. Their growth was fostered by the Hill-Burton program of 1954 and subsequently by Medicare and Medicaid. The first Medicare and Medicaid standards made nursing homes "skilled homes," and, according to Dunlop (1979), "significantly increased demand and costs and contributed to the use of skilled facilities for care that from a medical standpoint, at least, could be met in a less care intensive environment" (p. 101). In recognition of these developments, Congress established the Intermediate Care Facility (ICF) program under Title XI in 1967 and then included it under Medicaid funding in 1972. Prior to the level-of-care designations, regulation of nursing homes had been the exception rather than the rule.

Throughout the 1960s and 1970s, regulation of the nursing home industry grew. In response to reports of abuse, disasters, and increasing levels of public expenditures for nursing home care (Mendelson, 1974; Moss & Halamandaris, 1977), public attention to nursing homes and the quality of care provided there grew. Federal regulation and funding, however, such as the Hill-Burton program, focused attention on new facilities while "grandfathering" older, smaller facilities that were unlikely to be able to afford major structural improvements. In the early years, enforcement of regulations was difficult; few closures of facilities occurred because of lack of compliance. States had little funding to enforce the federal and state regulations, and the demand for nursing care was too great to implement policies that would limit the supply of homes available. It was not until 1974 that changes in federal Medicaid reimbursement provided the states 100 percent federal funding for all certification costs, thus allowing more effective enforcement of the regulations.

In addition, Medicare and Medicaid reimbursement levels for nursing home care were too low for facilities to meet all requirements and still serve older persons on public assistance (Dunlop, 1979). Throughout the 1970s, increasing regulatory requirements of staffing, fire safety, and personal and medical services contributed to the soaring costs of nursing home care. These made it more difficult for small facilities to compete in an environment in which they could neither take advantage of building loan programs nor benefit from economies of scale (Vladeck, 1980). Thus, more and more nursing homes became large, institutional environments, straying far from the nursing homes of earlier years that had more commonly been older, private homes adapted for this purpose and serving only a few older adults.

The history of the development and regulation of nursing homes and the policy trends evident in responses to the growth of the residential care industry have some critical similarities as well as differences. Specifically, it appears that the history of regulatory responses to the abuses seen in the nursing home industry has clearly shaped the recent policies that have developed to regulate residential care facilities. Figure 4.1, which highlights a few comparisons and contrasts in the regulatory responses in these two fields, provides an important framework for the review of current federal and state policies that affect residential care and for speculation on future developments in this changing field.

The history of public policy toward residential care can be compared to the policy that developed toward nursing homes. That is, public policy toward residential care

is largely a by-product of broader social welfare legislation, but in a tangential fashion. The history is like describing the opening of the American West from the perspective of mules; they were certainly there, and the epochal events were certainly critical to mules, but hardly anyone was paying very much attention to them at the time. (Vladeck, 1980, p. 31)

In much the same way that nursing home regulation developed, scandals in the residential care industry in the 1970s forced a policy response.

Figure 4.1
Comparisons/Contrasts: Growth of Regulatory Response in Nursing Homes and Residential Care Facilities

	NURSING HOME	RESIDENTIAL CARE
DEVELOPMENT OF POLICY ISSUE	Changing federal role in social welfare policies Response to scandals	Changing federal and state health care policies Response to scandals
REGULATORY GROWTH	Fueled by federal reimbursement	Not tied as closely to reimbursement as nursing home
FEDERAL INITIATIVE / OAA, 1953 / Keys, 1977	State responsibility Vague federal statute/state discretion in development of standards	State responsibility Vague federal statute/state discretion in development of standards
REGULATION	Initial focus on physical plant/later legislation "medicalizes" Focus on new facilities: older, small, home-like facilities often unable to meet standards Necessary to build larger, more institution-like homes to be profitable Prior to 1970, systematic inspections exception to the rule	Initial focus on physical plant, safety, staffing/ state legislation "medicalizes" Focus on new facilities: older small homes increasingly unable to meet standards Necessary to build larger, more institution-like homes to be profitable Prior to 1977, little or no inspection of homes for the aged, RCFs
ENFORCEMENT	Early years, 1964-66, no closures due to non-compliance Enforcement hampered because: Reimbursement is too low Demand for care is great Meager resources Enforcement enhanced by: 1974 – Changes in Medicaid for ICFs and 100% federal funding for certification costs made available to states	Early years, 1978–, no closures due to non-compliance. No enforcement of federal sanction Enforcement hampered because: Reimbursement is too low Demand for care is great Meager resources No enhancement for enforcement, no federal funding for surveys
OVERALL	Regulations changed from small, family-like settings to medical model, health care facilities	Potential for growth in regulations to change facilities from small, family-like settings to larger, more institution-like, health care settings

FEDERAL POLICY

Federal Response: The Keys Amendment

The 1976 Keys Amendment to the Social Security Act was the first of a series of federal initiatives resulting from increased pressure to provide for oversight of the board and care/residential care industry (Section 506[d] of P.L. 94–566, later to be designated Section 1616[e]). Originally introduced by Representative Martha Keys (Democrat, KS) as an amendment to H.R. 8911 (the SSI Amendments of 1975), this amendment largely came in response to concern lest the SSI program become a source of funding for substandard institutions. Only through the SSI funding channel could the federal government intervene in the oversight of these facilities. While the Keys Amendment did not provide for direct regulation of quality of care, life safety standards, or licensure for all facilities, "it attempted to stimulate state efforts to regulate and monitor board and care by requiring states to set and enforce standards concerning admission policies, life safety, sanitation, and civil rights protection for board and care facilities *where [significant numbers of] SSI recipients reside*" (Harrington et al., 1985, p. 178).

Not until January 31, 1978, were the regulations entitled "Standard-setting Requirements for Medical and Non-medical Facilities Where SSI Recipients Reside" (U.S. DHEW, 1978) issued. These regulations state that the purposes of the Keys Amendment were

> to assure development of standards for safe and appropriate residential settings as an alternative to institutional living for SSI recipients; 2. to limit the use of SSI funds for substandard facilities for such persons; and 3. to publicize the standards and enforcement procedures for these facilities as a means of involving the public in monitoring these standards. (U.S. DHHS, 1983, p. 54184)

As provided in the statute, states were required to

1. designate one or more state or local authorities to establish and enforce standards for residential facilities where significant numbers of SSI recipients reside or are likely to reside;
2. make annually available for public review a summary of the standards in the services plan under the former Title XX of the Social Security Act;
3. make available a list of any waivers of such standards and any violations that may have come to the attention of standard-setting authorities; and
4. certify annually to the Secretary of DHEW compliance with the Keys Amendment requirements. (U.S. DHHS, 1983, p. 54184)

Subsection (4), which authorized penalties for noncompliance, was the most controversial part of the amendment. It was the only enforcement provision contained in the Keys Amendment.

Payments made under this title with respect to an individual shall be reduced by an amount equal to the amount of any supplementary payment (as described in subsection [a] or other payment made by a state (or political subdivision thereof) which is made for or on account of any medical or any other type of remedial care provided by an institution of the type described in paragraph (1) to such an individual as a resident or an inpatient of such institution if such institution is not approved as meeting the standards described in such paragraph by the appropriate state or local authorities. (U.S. Public Law 94–566 Section 505[e], amending Section 1616[e] of the Social Security Act, 1976, p. 2687)

A separate provision of the Keys Amendment, amending Section 1611(e)(1)(c) of the Social Security Act, authorized SSI for eligible persons in small (no more than fifteen residents) publicly operated institutions (P.L. 94–566 Section 505[a]). A second federal initiative aimed at strengthening the state's ability to monitor and regulate board and care facilities came in a 1978 amendment to the Older Americans Act. This amendment recommended that nursing home ombudsman programs include advocacy for residents of board and care/residential care facilities (U.S. AOA, 1981).

Viewed from the historical perspective, the form in which the Keys Amendment developed is not surprising. Prior to 1935, the federal government played a minimal role in domestic policy. In colonial America, families and local government bore the responsibility for the aged and poor. The period from the Civil War until the Great Depression saw an increasing role of the federal government in areas formerly left to state control, but social welfare remained largely a state and local concern. However, "the enactment of the Social Security act marked the beginning of what has been termed cooperative federalism" (Lee & Benjamin, 1983, p. 66), with increasing federal involvement in at least the planning and administration of income support for the elderly and disabled.

The 1960s saw a second wave of federal expansion in social welfare policy, with the Great Society programs aimed at publicizing the extent of deprivation. In addition to programs aimed only at the poor, legislation such as the Older Americans Act was also included as part of a philosophy of concern for general public welfare. This era of categorical grants saw an increase in federal funding but at the same time focused on local control and the decentralization of planning. In spite of these changes, the basic structure of public assistance remained unchanged. The following decade saw the rise of Richard Nixon's "new federalism." Through programs such as revenue sharing and block grants, federal funds were provided to the states with as little federal involvement as possible. This trend continued under the Reagan administration and is perhaps best typified by the OBRAs of 1981 and 1987, which extended state discretion in the areas of social services and medical care under Medicaid.

The Keys Amendment can be viewed, then, as emerging from a body of welfare policy growing first out of the Elizabethan Poor Law and its embodiment in colonial America and then from the more recent attempts to define welfare policy delineated first in the Social Security Act of 1935. In particular, the passage of the Keys Amendment gave the states clear responsibility for setting licensure and certification standards within minimal, often vague guidelines set at the federal level. This approach is similar to the federal approach used in the original Title I, in SSI, and in the passage of Medicare and Medicaid. For example, under SSI, which affects the Keys Amendment, the states were allowed considerable discretion, through the option of supplementary payments or reimbursement, in the amount of assistance provided to low-income dependent populations. As with the legislation preceding it regarding old age policy, the Keys Amendment also made little realistic provision for enforcement.

The Keys Amendment can also be seen as a logical outgrowth of current theories of federalism and constitutional limitations on the power of federal and state governments. Specifically, policies and programs that affect the entire society more or less equally, such as national defense, are properly delegated to the federal government. Policies and programs that affect only one group of a society are appropriately assigned to local governments. It is thus assumed that local citizens can make decisions regarding the manner in which such programs will be implemented, given local fiscal constraints and policy priorities. This simplification of federalism overlooks the limitations on what local governments can do. They are limited in their ability to tax constituents, determine broader monetary policies, and control migration across their boundaries, limitations that may increase the demands for services offered within their jurisdiction. In addition, they are less able and less willing than the federal government to implement programs, such as social welfare, aimed at redistributive goals.

The first important trend to observe here is that most, if not all, of the social welfare policies that have dealt with the poor, the dependent, and the aged in the United States involve state discretionary policy; that is, responsibility is in the hands of the states (Estes, 1982). Thus: "The eligibility and benefits under these policies depend on the variable willingness and fiscal capacity of states to fund programs at the state level. . . . Not only are these state discretionary programs different from state to state; but they are easily politicized and are more economically vulnerable and variable than uniform federal policies" (Estes et al., 1983, p. 33). While some might argue that the structure of the policy implied by the Keys Amendment represents an attempt to promote a new policy style under the heading of new federalism (that is, legislation within a state-focused, federal cost containment philosophy), I would argue that more state discretion and responsibility are not new, nor are they tied to the concept of new federalism. They do reflect a general unwillingness, evident since the settlement of the country and continuing with the development of Social Security, for the federal government to assume responsibility for health and social welfare.

Second, in much the same pattern as the development of oversight for nursing homes, the legislative initiative came in response to scandals in the board and care arena, including catastrophes such as fires, and public outcry over reported abuses of residents. In Allison's model, the choices of how to counteract these catastrophes were framed by the organizational history and the routines built up within DHHS to respond to similar abuses in the nursing home industry, for example, regulation through reimbursement channels. DHHS, in turn, was constrained by the historical antecedents defining congressional responses to social welfare issues.

Impact of Organizational Framework. Examining DHHS as an organization within Allison's model demonstrates more fully the constraints on creative action. Allison described government organizations as often large, with a factored approach to problems in which aspects of the problems are parceled out to numerous suborganizations, each with its own sphere of power and influence. Federal programs for the aged clearly reflect this splintering of responsibilities. For example, the Administration on Aging is a separate agency within DHHS, operating independently of both the Health Care Financing Administration (HCFA), which administers both the Medicare and Medicaid programs, and the Social Security Administration, which administers the Old Age and Survivors Insurance Program and the Supplementary Security Income Program. It is also separate from the Department of Housing and Urban Development (DHUD), Veterans Administration, and the Departments of Labor, Transportation, and Agriculture, all of which administer programs affecting the elderly.

Responsibility for the Keys Amendment was even more ambiguous. In the original legislation, states were to report compliance to the Secretary of Health, Education and Welfare (HEW). No one agency within the organization was given responsibility for coordination. While the enforcement provision reflected the role of the Social Security Administration in identifying SSI recipients, no other agencies were given direct roles in program coordination. Responsibility for the 1978 amendment to the OAA, recommending advocacy for board and care residents under the nursing home ombudsman program, logically would fall to the Administration on Aging. This segmentation, and, in the case of the Keys Amendment, the lack of agency identification, has resulted in an inability to treat any major problem in a coherent fashion.

This tangle also reflects the confusion regarding residential care as a housing or care issue. Since no direct federal reimbursement for health care was involved, responsibility could not be assigned to HCFA. Since no funds or statutory guidelines were applicable under existing housing programs, DHUD was not involved. And while residential care was not really a nursing home, advocacy under the ombudsman program was seen as necessary. While many of the agencies within DHHS are involved in issues pertaining to residential care, none was directly charged with programs related to the Keys Amendment. This fact highlights another aspect of policy segmentation. Organizations frequently do not have jurisdiction over areas that are important to their assigned responsibilities or that are clearly related to areas in which they already have expertise.

At least theoretically, alternatives to these policy choices were available. An option could have been proposed that fell outside the medical model of health care and reimbursement employed in the nursing home field. The range of choices was limited, however, by existing organizational biases within DHHS and by agency capabilities. The philosophy of regulation that had developed in the field of nursing homes reigned, in spite of the fact that no direct federal reimbursement channels existed in the residential care industry through which control could be exerted. As Allison described it, the development of such regulations reflects the overriding propensity to approach problems as a reenactment of preestablished routines.

Given adequate funding and a willingness to work with other agencies, a creative approach to developing policy might have evolved through a joint effort among the Health Care Financing Administration, the Administration on Aging, and the other relevant departments within DHHS. DHUD, concerned with addressing the care needs of aging residents of 202 congregate housing units, could have been actively involved in delineating policy for the provision of assisted care in publicly subsidized facilities. Enforcement provisions might have been explored, using the existing ombudsman program, along with a critical review of the legal mechanisms outside the channels of federal reimbursement; some states had used them in dealing with nursing homes. As Bardach and Kagan (1982) have suggested, regulatory agencies might rely more than they do on educational strategies, mandatory disclosure regulations, or assistance to private litigants (p. 305) in addition to the use of existing avenues such as the ombudsman program. Yet existing organizational routines and political pressures to decentralize regulatory functions limited the range of creative responses.

The goals of the Congress and DHHS also limited the range of responses that could be considered. In Allison's model, responses that fit with existing organizational goals are more likely to be implemented. In an era in which the goal of cost containment was paramount, policy makers were caught between providing some mechanism for oversight while not penalizing a system that was providing cost-efficient care for many formerly institutionalized individuals. It cannot have escaped recognition, however, that the states were indeed "dumping" their institutionalized populations into facilities where the federal government, through SSI, would bear the cost of their supervision. These facilities were clearly providing care beyond bed and board. Some regulation was needed to insure the quality of the care already being provided, without turning the facilities into low-level nursing homes, complete with massive regulation.

Thus, the Keys Amendment emerged as a unique combination of state responsibility for the development of standards and a federal-based sanction for noncompliance. In their broadest application, however, this amendment and subsequent regulations provided for only minimal standard setting so as not to force the closure of scarce low-cost facilities. These regulations did not address problems in those private facilities providing care for middle- and upper-income residents who were not recieving SSI. Moreover, the amendment did not address the growing medical nature of these facilities.

These choices may be viewed as a trend away from "regulatory unreasonableness" (Bardach & Kagan, 1982, p. 6). While the regulatory approach to citizen protection has grown rapidly since the mid-1960s, both a political backlash and studies that strongly suggest that regulatory unreasonableness is an economic disincentive to the supply of goods and services have more recently curbed this growth. In the field of long-term care, excessive nursing home regulation has been cited as a significant factor in limiting the supply of nursing homes. In particular, nursing home regulation has made it more difficult for the smaller facilities to survive.

While few would argue against some regulation to insure the quality of care in facilities for the aged, disabled, and mentally impaired, the federal government has moved further away from strictly mandated federal schemes for compliance. Instead, recent programs have allowed state and local governments more discretion in setting standards for facilities and services, with the assumption that state-originated guidelines allow for more regional variation and are thus more "reasonable" to the majority of providers. Without federal criteria for evaluating the quality of care provided under the myriad state guidelines, however, most states have responded by drafting only process standards (for example, physical plant and staffing requirements) rather than the more difficult to measure performance standards (for example, quality of care measures).

It can be argued that a more comprehensive approach to the alternatives developing in the long-term care continuum is necessary. In the ideal scenario, such an approach might involve recommendations or standards issued by DHUD or DHHS for the design of new facilities and explicit requirements for the renovation and design of existing facilities to insure adequate fire and safety standards, as well as adaptive designs for impaired populations. This approach might also include requirements for the training of providers, which would necessitate the involvement of additional departments within DHHS. A comprehensive program for steering the industry might also include loan and special tax incentive programs through HUD, much as the Hill-Burton Act had provided an incentive for nursing home construction (Dunlop, 1979). A public education campaign, spearheaded jointly by older persons' advocacy groups and the Administration on Aging, could increase public awareness of this care alternative and focus attention on monitoring its quality and effectiveness in meeting the needs of consumers. As Allison pointed out, however, the prognosis for alternatives requiring such coordination among several organizations (and with groups outside the governmental structure) is poor. Such coordination would require some resolution of the housing versus care issue. No evidence exists that such alternatives were considered. The field of long-term care services is only beginning to address the overlapping nature of the programs and services provided for older persons.

In terms of Allison's model, the federal government, through DHHS, was also severely limited in its range of response by a lack of statutory authority. Most board and care facilities are privately owned; unlike nursing homes, there is no direct reimbursement to these facilities. Steeped in structuring regulation through the use of financial incentives/disincentives, DHHS devised a plan to urge states to effect standards for facilities where significant numbers of SSI recipients resided. In attempting to use this mechanism, however, the enforcement through reimbursement became a convoluted system aimed at recipients, not at providers. In effect, subsection (4) would punish violations of the law by reducing the SSI checks of residents in homes not in compliance with state regulation, including those states with no regulations at all. Clearly, this sanction did not seem in line with the intent of the amendment, which was to increase the number of low-cost, quality homes for low-income elderly, disabled, and mentally impaired.

In concept, states were to inspect and supervise board and care facilities and report violations to the Social Security Administration, which would, after giving appropriate notice, reduce the SSI payments of residents by the amount of supplement provided by a particular state or other state payment for medical or remedial care provided the resident by the home. It should be obvious that there was no incentive for states to report such violations, which would reduce an already scarce, low-cost resource within the community. In addition, the amendment provided no funds to states for training and salaries of inspectors.

The legislation was based on an incentive approach, assuming that if residents were informed that the facility in which they resided did not meet standards, they would move to another board and care home that had been approved under the regulations. As "consumers of care" they could take their SSI resources and purchase care in better quality homes that were meeting state requirements under implementation of the Keys Amendment. This approach is, in essence, a voucher system for purchasing residential care. Other federal programs that use a voucher approach to redistribution, such as rent subsidy experiments, have proven ineffective in ameliorating the problems of scarce or inadequate services. Other factors, including the large numbers who needed assistance, tight rental markets, and the lack of decent units available to low-income persons in many areas limited the program's effectiveness (Peterson, Rabe, & Wong, 1986).

In addition, such programs assume that those in need are capable of collecting information on the program and on facilities and are able to make clear and independent decisions based on this information. Such is clearly not the case for all recipients covered by the Keys Amendment. Many of them had been placed in residential care precisely because of their inability to exercise judgment and appropriate decision making.

The DHHS staff recognized the inequity of penalizing a recipient for the inadequacies of the facility, but it was unable to devise any alternative forms of enforcement. DHHS stated in the preface to the standard-setting regulations that it, along with Congress, intended to explore ways to amend the sanction subsection. Thus, even before implementation, organizational constraints had rendered a proposed programmatic guideline untenable.

Implementation at the Federal Level

Phase One. In an examination of implementation of the Keys Amendment, the first stage of the process in Rein's model—the development of guidelines—

is crucial, although one must keep in mind that the imperatives are at work at all stages. It is also important to remember that the constraints described in Allison's model on goal setting—special interests, organizational relationships, statutory authority, and others—are also at work at this stage of the process.

The rules and regulations for the implementation of Section 505 (d) of P.L., 94-566 were not issued until January 1978. In the development of these regulations, many special groups were consulted, including advocacy groups, state directors of human services, the national Governors Conference, and various bureaus in DHEW, including the Social Security Administration, the Administration on Aging, the Medical Services Bureau, the Children's Bureau, the Developmental Disabilities Office, and the President's Committee on Mental Retardation (U.S. DHEW, 1978). Since so many groups would potentially be affected by the ruling, it was essential to have input from as broad a spectrum as possible. In Rein's model, this participation may hamper consensus on the details of the guidelines but may also contribute to guidelines that seem more feasible to those who would implement the program at the state level. An examination of some issues on which direct input was solicited by DHEW may reflect accommodation between those affected groups (particularly the states) and the federal organization.

The law requires that standards be established for "any category of institutions, foster homes, or group living arrangements in which (as determined by the state) a significant number of recipients of SSI benefits is residing or likely to reside" (U.S. DHEW, 1978). Developers of the regulations were concerned with how "significant numbers of recipients" should be defined. The department expressed the belief that the states were in the best position to determine these definitions; the states responded positively. In addition, the department was concerned that all facilities, however small, follow the standards. Therefore, the regulatory guidelines indicated that the determining factor was not the number of SSI recipients living in a facility at any one time, but rather the likelihood or expectation that a significant number (which could be set as low as one person) would reside in the facility.

Input was also solicited by DHEW on the requirement that states publish summaries of their standards in their Title XX Social Services plan. States had expressed concern that where such regulations already existed and were published as administrative procedures in their states, additional publication would be a duplication of efforts. In this instance, the department felt that the additional publication was necessary to meet Title XX guidelines but that the summary need only be a listing of the items comprising the standards. In essence, a compromise was reached to reduce the workload for the states. Since the mechanism of the Title XX public review process had been used by the framers to inform and involve the public in standard setting, compliance with the Title XX guidelines was ruled necessary for full compliance.

Questions also arose between interested parties and the department over which kinds of facilities required standards and whether, instead of the penalty reducing recipients' benefits, some other sanction could be devised that would be directed at the substandard facility. In response to the first issue, it was not clear which facilities provided medical care and supervision, which were already certified for Medicaid and Medicare, and which provided only room and board. In an attempt to cover as many facilities as possible under the ruling, the department clarified by suggesting that Congress had expressed a distinct intent to have standards established for facilities that provide medical care, as well as any other category of institution. Facilities already certified for reimbursement under Title XIX of the Social Security Act were excluded, since the existing standards for participation in those programs exceeded the expectations for standards under the Keys Amendment. Facilities with only room and board were also to be excluded. In regard to the sanction provision, however, the department reaffirmed the intent of the legislation to reduce recipients' benefits as a means of reducing funds available to substandard facilities. Input from special interests and the states has been overwhelmingly negative ever since passage of the amendment, but no alternative has been put forth that seems feasible to the department. This provision continues to be a barrier to effective implementation and, while a source of contention, has never been enforced. It warrants further discussion here.

The legal imperative to enforce this aspect of the legislation has never been strong, because of the lack of belief in the sanction at all levels. Indeed, documentation prepared by the department and accompanying the regulations notes: "The Department recognizes the inequity of penalizing a recipient for the failings of the facility, and therefore intends to explore with Congress the possibility of amending the prescribed sanction. Comments are particularly welcome on the sanction itself and the Department's intention to seek to have it changed" (U.S. DHEW, 1978, p. 4017).

The inclusion of the sanction at all reflects the lack of knowledge and experience in regulation of facilities outside the federal reimbursement system and predicts its failure as an enforcement mechanism. Additionally, the rational-bureaucratic imperative implies that the mechanism will not be implemented by civil servants who do not accept it as a "reasonable and just" law. The compromise, then, is that state officials ignore the penalty provision and that DHHS ignores the complete lack of reported abuses. Subsequent amendments to the regulations and department efforts at improving implementation have yet to propose alternative sanctions and continue to stress the intent to preserve the sanction as written in the original mandate. (States also have other sanctions available at their own legislative discretion, such as civil and criminal penalties.)

Finally, the legislation permits the states to waive the standards under unique circumstances, which must be detailed and presented to the department as a request for waiver in each instance. This compromise allows the states some discretion in facilities peculiar to their region or service system, while final authority for inclusion remains with the federal agency charged with oversight.

In summary, the importance of the regulations that frame the implementation of the amendment cannot be overlooked. The legislation and subsequent regulations were intentionally ambiguous, leaving considerable discretion to the states in defining program guidelines. In light of the history from which the policy emerged, this ambiguity obviates the need for making clear value decisions in regard to the role and identity of residential care in the long-term care system; it permits numerous interpretations in the ambiguous areas. It is of interest that the department clearly recognized the lack of specificity in the law, stating that "the law is not specific on several important organizing and operational responsibilities integral to implementing Part 229 [Standard Setting Requirements for Medical and NonMedical Facilities Where SSI Recipients Reside]" (U.S. DHEW, 1978, p. 4019), including what types of state agencies would be appropriate for designation, how states would determine which kinds of facilities house significant numbers of SSI recipients, and where in the Social Security Administration reports of violations would be sent. Again, the department ruled that significant aspects of implementation were to be left to the discretion of the states. The states were given the choice of designating a responsible agency and were allowed to determine how to identify facilities, while violation reports were to be sent to regional Social Security offices. Perhaps the final and most critical variable determining the effectiveness of the regulation is the fact that the legislation provided no new funding to any state agency nor to the Social Security Administration for activities required by the law. In reference to Rein's model, this "environmental condition," an adequate level of resources required for action, is necessary for effective administration. As the discussion turns now to oversight and subsequent efforts to implement the provisions of the Keys Amendment more effectively, this variable remains crucial to the discussion.

Phase Two. Despite the intent of the Keys Amendment to encourage states to clarify their regulations (Stone et al., 1982), conditions in board and care and other residential facilities exhibited little improvement in the years immediately following its passage. Several studies (U.S. GAO, 1979; Mellody & White, 1979; Dittmar & Smith, 1983) have cited unsafe and unsanitary living conditions in facilities housing SSI recipients; they found that existing state regulations often excluded personal care and social needs, while focusing on the more evident and more clearly enforceable regulations governing physical features of the housing. This finding reflects what Bardach and Kagan (1982) have described as a focus on measurable rules. That is, rules are enforceable only if the enforcers can measure compliance. Certain "soft" variables, such as attitudes of caregivers and attention to social and psychological needs of residents, are more difficult to make subject to regulation.

In 1981, several fires in board and care facilities in New Jersey prompted Representative Matthew Rinaldo to write to the secretary of DHHS, Richard Schweiker. He urged a review of the implementation of the Keys Amendment to insure the protection of the increasing numbers of aged and disabled persons living in such residential facilities (Solomon, 1982). Subsequently, hearings were held through the U.S. Select Committee on Aging both to clarify the role of

DHHS in enforcement of the Keys Amendment and to highlight continued abuses in the industry.

A major focus of the hearings was the states' use of board and care facilities for emptying state-supported institutions. At one hearing, Representative Mario Biaggi stated that "in light of all these problems, our statistics show that the states are continuing to empty their institutions and to place the discharged individuals in boarding homes only after qualifying them with a Federal supplementary security income program" (U.S. Congress, 1981b, p. 2). In similar remarks, Representative Claude Pepper stated that there was a tremendous incentive for states to move people out of state mental institutions and place them in boarding homes, where the cost could be shifted to the federal SSI program (U.S. Congress, 1981a). Reports from the hearings also cited "widespread instances of poor living conditions and negligent care for a population which is, for the most part, indigent or elderly, and many of whom are former patients in mental institutions" (U.S. Congress, 1981b, p. 5).

The enforcement provision, subsection (4) of the amendment, continued to be controversial throughout the hearings. DHHS's witness at the hearings, David B. Swoap, Under Secretary of DHHS, stated that Secretary Schweiker had "clearly and emphatically rejected the notion of repealing the fourth provision of section 1616(e), with an eye toward working with Congress to develop amendments which will make it more workable, hopefully, and more directly address the problem at hand" (U.S. Congress, 1981b). DHHS, through Swoap, explicitly recognized the inequitable nature of the provision and its inadequacy as a corrective mechanism.

Following the congressional hearings, Secretary Schweiker requested that the inspector general (IG) conduct a study to identify the "best practices" of states in setting standards and regulating residential alternatives. Several changes affecting board and care homes occurred during the time of the IG's review that need to be noted.

First, OBRA of 1981 (U.S. P.L. 97–35) repealed the Title XX Social Services Program and enacted the Social Services Block Grant. This action effectively reduced federal funding and federal regulatory authority. In terms of the Keys regulations, it made unclear to which federal agency the states should send their summaries of the standards or their certifications of compliance. Second, the same act also gave DHHS the authority to grant home and community-based waivers under the Medicaid program; it declared that the states must provide assurances that the facilities used under the waiver met standards in certification. Third, the Rinaldo Amendment to the Older Americans Act was passed in December 1981, making mandatory the inclusion of board and care homes in a state's ombudsman program. These changes are the types of changes described by Rein as "oversight"; they incrementally contribute to changes in policy implementation.

The IG's report included several findings. First, widespread confusion existed over the distinction between boarding homes and board and care homes. Second, the report found evidence of continued low participation levels of states in oversight of board and care housing, including negligence in identifying facilities to be regulated; it did note the limitation placed on states by their lack of ability to close a facility that does not meet standards. Third, it cited a lack of leadership within DHHS for enforcement and implementation, a lack of coordination between the various components of the department that funded board and care research, and tardiness and lack of rigor in the final products of these various components (Kusserow, 1982).

Based on the recommendations of the report, the so-called "eight-point" program, outlined in April 1982, suggested that DHHS

1. establish a single unit in the Department with responsibility for providing Departmental leadership, and coordination of, board and care issues;
2. clarify procedures for state certification of compliance and publication of standards, in light of the block grant provisions affecting section 1616 (e);
3. consider establishment of a new sanction to give the Department leverage to enforce the requirements of the Keys Amendment;
4. grant Medicaid home and community based services waivers only to states certifying their compliance with the Keys Amendments;
5. establish greater protection against fraud for SSI board and care recipients in the SSI representative payee program;
6. increase technical assistance to the states;
7. develop a model state statute for board and care homes;
8. complete the development of fire safety standards for publication in the Life Safety Code. (Solomon, 1982, pp. 9, 10)

In Rein's model, the components of the oversight process, including monitoring, auditing, and evaluation, should act in a circular manner so that legislative intent is altered and administration modified as necessary to insure adequate implementation. The oversight hearings to review implementation of the Keys Amendment led to some clarification of the intent of the mandate (in particular, continued support of the sanction provision), the IG's report, and Schweiker's eight-point program. In turn, these activities did lead to changes in administrative practice.

As a result of the eight-point plan, the Board and Care Coordinating Unit (BCCU), administratively located in the Administration on Developmental Disabilities in the Office of Human Development Services, was established as the unit within DHHS responsible for implementing the plan. Some of the unit's initial activities provided funding during fiscal year 1982 for several research projects including:

1. a $390,000 grant to the National Bureau of Standards to complete the development of a Fire-Safety Evaluation System for board and care homes;
2. a $199,840 grant awarded to the National Fire Protection Association to conduct six seminars on fire-safety in adult boarding homes;

3. a grant of $98,769 to the New Jersey Department of Community Affairs to assist in the development of a management information system to be utilized in the regulation of board and care facilities; and
4. a $287,732 grant awarded to the American Bar Association to develop and disseminate model state statutory guidelines for regulation of board and care facilities. (U.S. DHHS, BCCU, 1983, p. 2)

In 1983, in response to continued need for clarification of the regulations governing implementation, DHHS issued a final rule on the Keys Amendment (U.S. DHHS, 1983). In response to comments, only one change was made in the regulations. That change allowed the states the option of charging a fee for providing copies of standards, procedures, or other regulations to the affected facilities. The additional comments accompanying the published final rule are of interest, however, in that they highlight the continued concern for the sanction provision, continued confusion over the types of facilities to be certified, and continued questions regarding what defines a "significant number" of SSI recipients. In response to OBRA, the rule also stipulated that all reports regarding compliance now be sent directly to the assistant secretary for Human Development Services. The ambiguous nature of the regulations necessitated the continuous definition and clarification of original intent. In practical terms, it has required numerous issuances from DHHS and has allowed many decisions to be made administratively, with limited public input.

In summary, while DHHS has attempted to clarify the federal role in insuring standards and quality of care to board and care residents, the intent has not been fulfilled in many cases. Among the barriers to implementation that may account for this lack of success are

1. inadequate resources available to states to pay for the licensing and inspection of all board and care homes;
2. the problems of identifying unlicensed board and care homes;
3. lack of funds to pay for improved care in board and care homes (There is little margin in the basic SSI payment to pay for services after an allowance for basic board and lodging.);
4. the difficulties of coordinating and managing the different agencies responsible for providing support and services to disabled and aged persons living in the community; and
5. uncertainty as to what standards are appropriate for board and care homes. (U.S. DHHS, BCCU, 1983, p. 3).

Lack of funding has been perhaps the most crucial variable in the implemention of the Keys Amendment. Because no additional federal funds have been made available for the activities required, the burden has fallen on the states to create strategies using existing scarce resources to implement regulatory and monitoring programs. In addition, any efforts taken to regulate the industry can have an impact on the supply of suitable housing. In spite of these obstacles, many states have undertaken expansion of their regulatory and monitoring functions, providing further protection for residents in these residential facilities.

CHAPTER 5

The Oregon Experience

Like other states, Oregon began to expand its regulation and monitoring of the residential care industry following the passage of the Keys Amendment. Oregon differed from some states, however, in that some expansion of monitoring functions predated the Keys Amendment. The need to comply with the Keys Amendment provided the impetus to develop standards for facilities and care further and provided Oregon a measure by which to compare its previous efforts.

This review of Oregon's experience in residential care used several methods of data collection. Sources include state archival records, individual staff records from state departments, state administrative rules and staff manuals, and interviews with administrators, planners, program supervisors, and staff involved in monitoring residential care facilities or in placing clients in residential care throughout the state.[1] Based on this array of information, this chapter analyzes Oregon's experience in implementing the Keys Amendment. This chapter reviews the conceptual issues, the demand and supply factors, the history of residential care definitions and regulations in Oregon, and the current regulatory responses.

CONCEPTUAL ISSUES AND HISTORICAL INFLUENCES: HOUSING OR CARE

Before the late 1960s, Oregon had followed the example of the rest of the nation, allowing board and care homes and homes for the aged to operate with little or no regulation. Since the passage of stringent nursing home regulations, these facilities had offered a less expensive alternative to nursing home care and provided (at least in theory) care for a somewhat healthier population who needed only minimal supervision. Between the late 1960s and 1977, "homes for the aged" were licensed by the state Health Division. At first glance, the placement of these facilities within the purview of the Health Division in the late 1960s implies that policy makers were concerned with the medical care aspects of these facilities. According to one state staff member, however, it reflected more a concern with cleanliness standards, similar to those applied to restaurants and other public facilities. Board and care facilities and homes for the aged were still considered primarily a housing option for older people. Only minimal standards existed; the renewed licenses were often automatically mailed to the facilities upon their expiration date. Few surveys were done. They were undertaken only when a serious problem was reported.

The earliest evidence of increasing concern with board and care facilities can be found in a bill drafted in 1973 by the Board and Room Association that would have addressed many of the concerns subsequently covered by SB 100. Although the first bill was defeated, a licensing bill, HB 3056, was passed. Its standards (ORS 443), administered through the Health Division, took effect on January 11, 1975, and were implemented by 1977. These standards did not cover room and board facilities but did address homes for the aged and group care homes. They reflected a growing recognition of the personal and medical care being provided in these settings.

Until 1977, facilities that provided nonnursing care to persons 65 years of age or older were defined by the Oregon State Health Division as Homes for the Aged (HAs) or Sheltered Care Homes (Oregon Administrative Rules, CH. 333, effective November 15, 1974). House Bill 3056 clearly made these homes separate from those facilities serving the mentally and physically handicapped. The new law defined group care homes as distinct from HAs or sheltered care homes and required that the Health Division, in cooperation with other affected state departments, developed rules for group care homes.

Under the Health Division guidelines, an HA was defined as a "facility which furnishes food, shelter, and personal services for compensation to three or more residents not related by blood or marriage and excludes persons who are completely bedfast or persons requiring nursing care" (OAR, Section 23–550, [5], March 1975, p. 1). Domiciliary care or personal services, in contrast, were defined as "services which emphasize supervision, protection, and assistance while bathing, dressing, eating, grooming, and administering medication and directed toward self-care skills of the resident" (OAR, Section 23–550, [3], March 1975, p. 1).

These rules provided for licensure, outlined rules for administrative management (including guidelines for the types of residents who could be served), and set staffing requirements. At that time, a registered nurse was required to be on call at all times, but no experience or professional training was required of the on-site attendant. Minimum attendant coverage was defined as "1 attendant for every 20 residents or major fraction thereof" for both day and evening shifts and 1 attendant "up and dressed" (p. 4) for every 40 residents during the night shift. Standards were set for the residents' environment, including minimal space requirements per resident bed and toilet and bath ratios. General guidelines were also outlined for resident care and activities; more specific regulations were detailed for dietary services, medical records, pharmaceutical services, and sanitation practices.

In an attempt to address the fiscal concerns of small home providers (fewer than twenty residents), the staffing requirements were amended as of May 24, 1976. This amendment changed the night shift requirements in facilities with one through twenty residents to allow for "an electrical call system in each resident room terminating in an attendant's sleeping area" in lieu of an attendant up and dressed. In addition, facilities of more than twenty residents still had to provide one attendant up and dressed during the night shift; facilities of over fifty residents required two attendants up and dressed; and one additional attendant up and dressed was required for each major fraction over fifty residents (Memo, Oregon State Health Division–Health Facilities Licensing and Certification [OSHD-HFLC], June 1, 1976).

These early regulations have interesting similarities to those governing nursing homes. Clearly, the state looked to its experience in the regulation of nursing homes in drafting the guidelines for homes for the aged. Staff ratios, rules governing personal care, and administration of medications all are based on a medical model of care. Yet staff members in recent interviews report that no one during the 1970s would have referred to homes for the aged as medical care settings. This lack of clarity regarding the nature of residential care settings allowed these original regulatory attempts to acknowledge care needs without requiring extensive intervention in the facilities.

STATE RESPONSE

Increased Regulatory Intervention: Senate Bill 100

While the existing regulations covered many aspects of operation, they were very general and provided for only a minimum of oversight. They did not address the growing medical nature of the care provided, the need for more stringent fire safety regulations, or the skills and training needed by providers. It is useful, however, to compare the regulations existing at this time for HAs with those for group care homes, which served primarily the mentally and physically impaired.

Regulations governing group care homes (OAR, Sections 23–500 through 23–538) held more stringent guidelines for (1) determination of the ability of residents to respond to fire or other emergency; (2) resident evaluation and case management; (3) staff training, including orientation and in-service requirements; (4) medication records; (5) physical environment; and (6) resident training and activities. In addition, staffing requirements were greater than those required by HAs, with group homes requiring one staff person for fifteen residents. State reimbursement for homes for the aged was commensurately less than that for group homes. Even in 1978 the figures reflected this difference, with homes for the aged receiving $92 per resident per month, while group homes received $215–$323 per resident per month.

These fiscal inequalities, the growing confusion between providers and state governmental units about inspection and regulation, and the need for more detailed regulations in all aspects of residential care led to the passage in 1977 of Senate Bill 100 (SB).

SB 100 can be seen as the product of proposals put forth during 1976 by an interdivisional group of the Department of Human Resources (DHR). This group, including representatives from the Mental Health Division, the Health Division, the Corrections Division, the Children's Services Division, and the Public Welfare Division, met for eight months during 1976. With assistance from a representative of the Fire Marshal's Office, the group produced recommendations for changes in the residential care industry. Their findings and recommendations were then submitted to provider and consumer groups during the months of October and November 1976. While the final draft of these changes, represented by SB 100, was not fully acceptable to all, most concerns were incorporated into the final draft.

The bill, introduced at the request of DHR, represented an attempt to resolve inconsistencies, ambiguities, and confusion regarding the regulation of residential facilities. Simply put, the bill combined existing licensing statutes relating to group care homes and HAs and transferred supervision over such facilities from the Health Division to the department level.

During the first consideration of the bill by the Senate Committee on Aging and Minority Affairs (January 15, 1977), Bob Oliver, then deputy director of the Department of Human Resources, told the committee that

SB 100 relates to nonmedical residential care homes and facilities and reflects an attempt to identify those areas where two or more divisions are involved in the administration of the same program and their efforts overlap, gaps exist between jurisdictions, and/or directions and policies are not well coordinated. (Oregon State Senate, 1977a, p. 1)

In addition, Oliver stressed to the committee that SB 100 "is not intended to impose stringent new requirements on any facilities; it is intended to consolidate management responsibilities which will work more effectively in the interests of the clientele and the industry itself" (p. 1). The Measure Intent Statement accompanying the bill further clarified the intended function of SB 100. It declared that the function and purpose of the measure as reported were the following:

1. Give the Department of Human Resources and its director greater flexibility in the administration of and setting standards for various kinds of group care homes.
2. Transfer supervision over residential care homes and facilities from the Health Division of the State Department of Human Resources to the department generally.

3. Specify the size of group care home, which in some cases, would make possible lower cost of operation. (Oregon State Senate, 59th Legislative Assembly, Measure Intent Statement–SB 100)

Several issues raised before the Senate Committee during the initial January 15, 1977, meeting should merit attention. Testimony was provided by several special interest groups, including the Coalition of Senior Advocates, Oregon Residential Facilities Association, Christian Science Committee on Publication, and Marion County Chapter of Oregon Association for Retarded Citizens, and by staff from the Department of Human Resources, Public Welfare Division. They expressed concern over the implications of the new facility definitions, the appeals process for providers, issues surrounding the training component, and the omission of statutes to govern adult foster care for the elderly.

Definitions. SB 100 provided new definitions for residential facilities. Specifically, the bill separated those facilities providing training from those providing care. The definitions included in the bill read:

1. "Residential training facility" means a facility that provides, for six or more mentally retarded or other developmentally disabled individuals, residential care and training in one or more buildings on contiguous properties.
2. "Residential treatment facility" means a facility that provides, for six or more mentally, emotionally or behaviorally disturbed individuals, residential care and treatment in one or more buildings on contiguous properties.
3. "Residential care facility" means a facility that provides for six or more physically handicapped or socially dependent individuals, residential care in one or more buildings on contiguous properties. (SB 100, Section 1, [6, 7, 8], p. 1)

This change was critical to those in mental health, where the previous rule defined a group care home as a facility that provided care, boarding, *and* training. The mandatory inclusion of training had been a difficult requirement for many group homes to meet without additional revenues or reimbursement. It did not necessarily apply to homes serving the aged or the mentally, emotionally, or behaviorally disturbed. The new definitions thus recognized the differences among treatment, training, and care and thereby reduced the requirements for some types of group homes. The definitions also gave group homes the option of providing care to a broader spectrum of clients, including the aged. In addition, the choice of six or more residents for inclusion under the new law was consistent with the fire marshal's regulations. Interestingly, SB 100 did not specifically mention the elderly or aged in the definition but provided the term *socially dependent.* With this focus on social dependency, the omission again reflected the continued lack of clarity regarding the social or medical nature of these facilities.

The administrative rules that followed SB 100 implicitly made further distinction between residential care homes and residential care centers. Anna Helm of DHR noted that this distinction would be used in the new rules in an effort to "enhance and emphasize a residential setting rather than an institutional environment" (Senate Committee on Aging & Minority Affairs, January 25, 1977, Exhibit "6"). A residential care home would serve at least six but fewer than sixteen individuals, while a residential care center would serve sixteen or more individuals. This change also allowed for distinct rules to be written for each, taking into account the impact of physical plant requirements and care provision in smaller versus more institutional settings. The distinctions included in the Oregon rule illustrate the array of definitions of residential care that makes cross-state comparison so difficult. Ironically, the change in definition was intended to clarify residential care, with the "care" category taking the place of the old homes-for-the-aged rules. Unfortunately, Mental Health also had facilities that it thought should come under "care." As one state staffer noted, "We wound up with all these confusing issues about the different kinds of care facilities."

Sanctions. Amid controversy, the bill strengthened sanctions. Section 12 of SB 100, which detailed circumstances under which a facility license could be revoked or suspended, came under question by Charles Lawson of the Oregon Residential Facilities Association (Senate Committee on Aging & Minority Affairs, January 25, 1977, Exhibit "1"). Specifically, in the case where a resident has been removed because of wrongdoing on the part of a home, Lawson's organization requested a provision to allow the home to appeal revocation or suspension to some independent board or commission not directly involved in licensure. This provision, he believed, would reduce the necessity of the owners' seeking redress through litigation. The final bill included no such provision. (A public appeals process does exist in accordance with OAR, Chapter 183, Administrative Procedures Act, which governs appeals and all other licensing laws.)

In addition, the Oregon legislature adopted a measure in 1975 authorizing the administrator of the State Health Division to impose civil penalties on nursing homes violating state laws or rules prescribing minimum standards. Section 13 of SB 100 authorized the director of DHR to exercise similar authority regarding residential facilities. The inclusion of this section provided a mechanism for enforcing compliance beyond that provided by the Keys Amendment. Again, Lawson objected to the types of penalties that could be levied under this section. Specifically, his testimony stated that "we are concerned that medical model penalties for minor or major infractions of rules are not the penalties needed for a social model facility" (p. 5).

The housing versus care issue had thus arisen on a public level. In his testimony, Lawson provided a brief historical overview that contributes some insight. As he noted, the Oregon Residential Facilities Association had worked diligently to define what it saw as a clear distinction between group care homes, "those based on a social model, where the goal was a normal environment, a place to be trained, and a place to work toward the prevention of further handicaps or as an alternative to nursing care" (p. 2) and HAs, which he grouped with nursing homes and hospitals under the medical model. In his words, "the medical and social models were continually being confused with one another by those who requested compliance with the rules" (p. 3).

HAs (or, now, residential care homes) were promoted by professionals as nonmedical, community alternatives for elderly people. Statute and the attitudes of providers, however, continued to support a medical model for such facilities if they focused on an aged population. When they served a younger, mentally impaired population, they were seen as facilities based on a social model. I would argue that SB 100 did little to clarify this issue and in fact paved the way for the further "medicalization" of residential facilities for the aged.

Obvious Omissions. The bill also omitted from its province foster homes for adults and room and board situations. George Corwin of the Coalition of Senior Advocates questioned this omission (Senate Committee on Aging & Minority Affairs, January 25, 1977, Exhibit "2"). Lucille Pugh, DHR program manager, Adult Service Section, answered by submitting a copy of administrative rules with reference to approval of foster homes for adults prepared by the Public Welfare Division (Senate Committee on Aging & Minority Affairs, January 25, 1977, Exhibit "5"). These rules aimed to protect individuals, both elderly and disabled, in homes caring for five or fewer residents; they thus covered those facilities not defined by SB 100. It is of interest that while foster homes have become the fastest growing form of alternative care for older people in Oregon, particularly for those on state assistance, policy makers did not deem them appropriate to protect or regulate by direct statute. Instead, regulation was left to administrative rule through various departments. State statute has since provided for foster homes.

Final Passage. A second Senate committee hearing was held on February 15, 1977, and its brief discussion focused on amendments to address the issues raised by various groups in the January meeting. Following this discussion, the committee voted to move SB 100 to the floor with a "Do pass as amended" recommmendation. The Senate Ways and Means Committee reviewed SB 100 on April 4, with special attention to the fiscal impact of the bill. Statements prepared by the Legislative Fiscal Office (February 15, 1977; April 1, 1977) had shown the impact of SB 100 to be minimal, projecting additional revenue from the increase in licenses issued and renewed per biennium at $50 each. These projected increases in revenue fell from an original figure of $6,870 to a revised figure of $3,485 (for fiscal years 1977-79).

Interestingly, the potential fiscal impact of combining HAs and group care homes, which had previously had widely disparate funding levels, was not addressed at this time, nor was the cost of staff needed to implement SB 100 adequately. These and other fiscal issues arose during implementation when the administrative rules were formulated. The omission of additional funds needed to carry out the intent of SB 100 has continued to inhibit the effectiveness of the regulatory agencies. The initial fiscal vagueness was a necessary political maneuver on the part of DHR to avoid any additional discussions of potential fiscal impact that might have jeopardized passage of the legislation.

SB 100 continued to the House for review, with many of the same concerns addressed, including clarification of definitions and the civil penalties section. Specifically, John Richard of the Oregon Health Care Association noted that the penalties were designed for nursing homes and were not necessary for residential care (House Committee on Aging, April 21, 1977, Minutes, p. 2). DHR had supported the inclusion of Section 13 on the rationale that agencies were less likely to prosecute for criminal penalties (provided under Section 14) than for civil penalties; less action would be taken if criminal penalties were the only recourse. The section was therefore included as an "extra remedy" for insuring compliance (Bob Oliver, DHR, House Committee on Aging, April 21, 1977, Minutes, p. 3). During this House committee meeting, however, Oliver noted DHR's willingness to wait until the bill had been in place for one year to see if this section would be necessary in order to insure swift passage of the bill.

In a second meeting of the committee on May 5, 1977, Representative Mary Burrows objected to an amendment presented by Ted Hughes of the Oregon Health Care Association to delete the civil penalty (Exhibit C, SB 100 − #2). Following some discussion no further action was taken on the sanction provision. SB 100 was thus sent to the House Ways and Means Committee with a "Do pass" recommendation and was then reported to the House with a "Do pass as amended" recommendation on June 17, 1977. SB 100 was passed by the House on June 23 and by the Senate on June 24, 1977, to become effective July 1, 1978 (SB 100, Section 26).

Summary: Regulation within Frameworks. In summary, SB 100 was clearly not a direct response to the Keys Amendment, a response that came later in 1978. State policy makers anticipated, however, many of the areas that would have to be addressed. Within the Allison and Rein models described earlier, the passage of SB 100 shows both similarities and some marked differences to the Keys Amendment history.

Unlike the federal response, the state bill came out of the regulatory divisions themselves, in response to direct needs seen by the staff. Although abuse had been documented in homes for the aged, the impetus for change came less from direct catastrophes, the public, or political motivations of state representatives than from those within the state divisions who recognized the inadequacy of existing guidelines to monitor and regulate this rapidly growing field of care. In addition, some impetus came from providers who questioned the applicability of existing rules, particularly those involved in mental health care in group homes.

This type of policy change can be seen as an example of the "rationalizing politics" suggested by Brown (1983b). In contrast to what might be termed "breakthroughs," Brown has argued that rationalizing politics more clearly represents the way in which current policies are defined. Using recent examples in health care reform (such as the launching of health maintenance organizations) and regulation of the airline and trucking industries, Brown asserted:

That these initiatives were enacted not because of widespread constituency support, critical realignments, or party platforms, but instead largely as a result of government's own discontent with the workings of earlier governmental programs, suggests that there is a new and important political mode—rationalizing politics—which the deadlock-breakthrough syndrome [characterizing earlier policy developments] does not describe well. (P. 11)

State legislators were constrained in the development of SB 100 by previous experience, as were those within DHR involved in the design of the Keys Amendment. Their reliance on previous rules regarding group homes and homes for the aged and their reliance on the nursing home model for the sanction provision limited the range of alternatives considered. On the one hand, the reliance on existing organizational routines and policies may be seen as a positive evolution, whereby the divisions build upon previous experience, continuing to refine policy as changes occur in both the political sector and the industry itself. On the other hand, as Allison notes, this reliance may limit creativity when something more than incremental change is needed.

In regard to the sanction provision, the state faced a dilemma similar to that faced by framers of the Keys Amendment. That is, it was important to have an effective sanction for insuring compliance, yet the options for "do-able" sanctions were limited. The state, perhaps more clearly, recognized that a "market approach" to sanctioning, that is, assuming that clients would move from inappropriate or inadequate facilities, was not a realistic expectation; nor was the closure of facilities, accomplished through the revocation of licenses, in the best interest of the clients. Thus, the reliance on the civil penalties section was incorporated with the ability to levy financial penalties or other sanctions on providers in order to insure compliance.

Perhaps most importantly, SB 100 was left intentionally vague through statute, much like the Keys Amendment, with the charge to the Department of Human Resources to draft administrative rules for implementing the statute. While Rein acknowledged the importance of the guideline development process in determining policy at the national level, I believe that this process is perhaps an even more critical policy stage at the state level. State policy covers more specific day-to-day operations of services and facilities and must be outlined in great detail to insure coordination of all departments involved in monitoring and regulation. At the state level, this tangle of regulations has perhaps been most obvious with Medicare and Medicaid, in which cases the states must implement a confusing array of federal regulations within their own state guidelines. With the passage of SB 100, the process of rules development had particular importance, for it became the stage for providers to express again their concerns with the legislation.

Implementation: Administrative Rules and the Keys Amendment

Task Force. Immediately following adjournment of the legislature in 1977, the SB 100 Task Force was organized and charged with developing and recommending administrative rules and licensing procedures to implement SB 100. The task force was divided into committees, one for each type of facility defined by the statute. There were thus committees on training facilities, on treatment facilities, and on care facilities. These committees focused on what care would be provided and how it would be monitored. In addition, a Committee on Licensing Procedures and other issues common to all facilities, including fire and safety issues, was formed as the fourth standing committee (Mental Health Division Memo, SB 100 Status Report, June 16, 1978).

As stated in the Memo of June 16, 1978, the major objectives of the task force were the following:

1. Develop new license application and issuance procedures;
2. Develop rules that centralize license application process into a "one step" process;
3. Take action on license application within 30 days;
4. Use existing technical expertise within state agencies for on-site review and approval of license applications;
5. Maintain a "current status" file on all licenses;
6. Activate existing technical expertise within state agencies to address issues of license suspension and revocation;
7. Activate existing technical expertise within state agencies to renew existing licenses;
8. Define specific roles for each state agency in licensing and monitoring procedures;
9. Develop new Administrative Rules as required by Section 6 (2) of S.B. 100;
10. Complete all requirements for implementing S.B. 100 by July 1, 1978;
11. Develop rules and procedures that are implementable within existing agency resources;
12. Include as participants in rules and procedures development process representatives of major groups and agencies that will be impacted by the outcomes;
13. All rules developed shall be in the same format and use common language and requirements.

Item 11 is of particular concern in examining the outcomes of the committee process. As noted by one state employee serving on a committee, "The fiscal impact was the foremost thing in our minds when working on the committees because when we thought something should be included, we would have to consider whether there was fiscal impact either to the agencies or the providers, and essentially we were told there could be none." This constraint was to have important effects.

The Keys Amendment was passed in 1977, just after the task force began to meet; the standards issued by DHHS were issued on January 31, 1978. The state committees now had to consider these federal mandates as well in designing the regulations. While the Keys Amendment did not outline specific requirements in the areas of fire safety, sanitation, resident rights, and quality care, it did encourage the states to develop standards in these areas and did provide for reducing or withholding SSI assistance payments from recipients as a sanction for inadequate care. The state of Oregon was already working on the rules, and, as one staff member said, "We had just filed our first rules for foster care at the time the Keys Amendment started being required . . . so, we felt pretty smug about the fact that we were ahead of the game at that point." The state thus had to consider primarily how to locate all facilities housing SSI recipients and how to complete the certification process to verify that compliance was in order.

Interestingly, the committees labored over what the Keys requirements meant by "significant numbers of SSI recipients." One source reported that DHHS considered one or more a significant number; because the state licensing regulations already included the care component of the facilities and defined the numbers in each type of facility, the state (committees) decided that they were meeting the requirement.

Throughout 1978 the committees developed the administrative rules and licensing procedures. They hoped that all new rules would be finalized by November. By the middle of 1978, however, it became obvious that many facility licenses would come up for renewal before the complete rules and procedures were finalized. Thus, effective August 8, 1978, DHR filed Administrative Rule 410–04–002 as a temporary rule pertaining to licensing. It provided that all residential care, treatment, and training facilities should be licensed for a two-year period, as opposed to the previous one-year license policy, and applied a flat $50 fee to all applications. Previously, these fees had varied by type and size of facility. The temporary rule stipulated that rules existing prior to SB 100 pertaining to civil penalties, health, sanitation, programs, and other issues would remain in effect until the new rules could be completed.

Following the filing of the temporary rule, a draft of the permanent rule on licensing was sent to the divisions for formal fiscal impact review. A more accurate picture began to emerge of at least one area of fiscal impact of SB 100 on the state divisions involved. For example, the division's estimates of the shortfall expected as a result of reclassifying homes for the aged and group care homes ranged from $7,000 to $15,000. These changes in revenue resulted from (1) less frequent licensing and changes in the fee structure (SB 100, Sections 8 [1] and 9 [1]); and (2) the transfer of monies collected from the Health Division to the Department of Human Resources (SB 100, Section 10 [2]). These changes implied that the Health Division would lose not only the application for licensure fees but also possible fees derived from the Civil Penalties Section (13) or Class B Misdemeanor Section (14).

In addition, DHR would need more staff to implement the additional work required by the rules; the fiscal impact on providers would change if the new regulations were passed in their various draft forms. No additional staff was to be provided to DHR, however, except that the registered nurse who had been doing the surveys within the Health Division would move to DHR, initially on a contract basis. Fiscal impact on providers was potentially large, for example, in meeting increased fire safety regulations, providing increased medical and dental coverage, and adapting new physical plant requirements for dining and activity space. In fact, one memo, dated October 18, 1978, stated that if the rules were implemented as they were presently written, additional funds in the amount of $3,860,935 would be needed. Additional funds at this level were inconceivable, so the administrative staff of DHR recommended deleting or amending those draft regulations that showed considerable fiscal impact and adopting those that did not.

The Care Committee had also been working through various drafts of its rules during 1978. These rules were reviewed by providers and staff. In 1979, the final proposed rules, with some (for example, mandatory dental evaluations and yearly dental visits for all residents) deleted or amended to reduce fiscal impact, were mailed to interested parties for final review. This mailing list represented a range of public and private interests, including such groups as the Oregon Residential Care Association, Association of Retarded Citizens, Western Association of Health Care Providers, Oregon Association of Homes for the Aged, and involved state divisions, such as the Fire Marshal's Office.

In addition, hearings on the rules were held throughout the state to allow for further input before their filing on July 26, 1979. The rules were then prepared for final distribution to be included in Volume III of the Oregon Adult and Family Services (AFS) Staff Manual (AFS, Manual Letter, III–102, August 8, 1979). Additional rule modifications were distributed in 1980, clarifying the licensure process, defining the responsible party within AFS for inspections and licensing, and incorporating the revised DHR Administrative Rules regarding Adult Residential Care Homes and Centers, effective September 9, 1980. At this time, Adult and Family Services Division officially took over responsibility for licensing and surveying residential care homes and centers from the Health Division.

Some comments from providers during the period of review were especially interesting. Primarily, the providers expressed concern with the growing medical nature of residential care as reflected in the proposed rules. Here is a lengthy quotation from a letter to the Task Force from Martha Scharpf, administrator:

Homes for the Aged are a viable alternative to nursing care for a great many people now being cared for in nursing homes. The reimbursement level between the two differs markedly. And, incidentally, the reimbursement level for HA is unrealistically low, given the demands which will now be made upon them. . . . What is happening now, however, is the development of a new set of rules where the medical model with its demands for record-keeping, close supervision, and staff is going to create a fiscal impact that will force the Homes for the Aged to un-license or close. . . . Residential Care should be just that. . . . The real value of Residential Care is that it creates a safe environment and *does not* meet medical or nursing needs. . . . If the need is for nursing, let it be given in that setting. If it is retirement and residential care, allow residents to function without constriction. . . . When committees seek to develop Rules, the implication is to assume complete control. If that happens to Homes for the Aged, you have lost the point of their existence and added immeasurably to State costs by increasing reimbursement, more staff to survey, and pushing persons faster into nursing services. (Letter to Lu Dethlefs, Program Coordinator, June 23, 1978)

This letter poignantly describes the confusion between housing and care that existed, and still exists, in the field of residential care. While the new rules still assumed a largely ambulatory population, some of the proposed requirements, and those subsequently implemented, for resident care reflected a changing orientation from supervision to care. Yet certain medical care requirements were omitted, reflecting the confusion regarding the care function.

A review of some of the major changes brought by SB 100 and the new regulations (Administrative Rule, Ch. 410) may clarify the problem.

Implementation: Conceptual Areas Addressed

Fire Safety. Unlike the homes for the aged, residential care homes would now have to identify the "self-preservation level" of residents to be served. This requirement related to the mandatory fire safety standards, which stated that the home must provide fire safety equipment appropriate to the number and level of residents served. Roughly, these levels include I–1, the highest level of protection, required by nursing homes; I–2, where some assistance is needed by residents to vacate the building in an emergency (most residential care facilities); I–4 (now SR–1), where residents are totally ambulatory. (SR–1 is a designation for "Special Residential," applies largely to very small homes, and modifies the standards somewhat for their size.) The regulations mandated that, within thirty days from time of admission, the facility must determine each resident's ability to depart from the building when warned by a signal device. For those facilities with I–2 and I–4 status, the regulations now required such improvements as sprinklers and hard-wire ionization. By requiring that specific resident levels be determined, the fire safety standards for residential care improved significantly.

Building Requirements. The new regulations mandated for the first time a specific amount of common space for each resident, 15 square feet per resident, in addition to the minimum 60 square feet per resident of bedroom space. The ratio of showers per resident also increased, with one bathtub or shower required for each ten residents (versus fifteen in the old HA rules). This change reflected the assumption that most residents would be ambulatory and that residential care should vary from the nursing home model to some extent.

Admission/Discharge Policies. In entirely new sections, the regulations spelled out specific guidelines for admission and discharge for residential care and mandated that a plan of care for each resident be developed within one week of admission. This rule in particular might be seen as reflecting the move to a more medical model of care provision, but a specific care plan had been required for group care homes (Mentally Retarded/Developmentally Disabled [MRDD]; Mentally and Emotionally Disabled [MED]) and for nursing homes for some time. The rule was thus clearly an attempt to determine the specific types of care being given to residents in residential care facilities.

These new rules allowed residents to receive notice at least fourteen days in advance of a move or transfer; they also required a facility staff meeting to review the appropriateness of the move and to coordinate services needed by the resident following the move. This clause provided protection for those residents who might be moved without due process because of their difficult behavior, financial difficulties, or incompatibility with the administrator or other residents.

Residents' Rights. Section 18–100 clearly defined residents' rights based largely on the nursing home Bill of Rights currently in use in long-term care.

Resident Activities. The new regulations outlined specifically what the resident activities should include and required that facilities develop a volunteer program to "promote resident participation in community centered activities." Perhaps most important, the new regulations required that transportation for medical services be arranged by the facility. This requirement did not mean that facilities would have to provide the transportation; it meant that they would have to assist the resident in obtaining transportation for needed medical care.

Health Services. The new regulations significantly increased the medical documentation required for each resident and placed more stringent guidelines on medication supervision. Interestingly, the old HA rules required that facilities have a registered nurse consultant on call at all times. In reviewing the new regulations, most providers felt that the nurse consultant was not needed since the staff had to go to the physician anyway for medication and treatment orders. Therefore, the DHR staff omitted this requirement from the new regulations. This change indicated the ambivalence felt by both providers and staff regarding the medical needs of residents. As a registered nurse from the state noted, these less stringent regulations perhaps reflected the more ambulatory nature of the residents at that time. At the same time, however, other changes in the regulations were aimed at providing a more medical model of documentation and care.

Staffing. Staffing requirements for residential care homes versus residential care centers (those with sixteen or more residents) were clarified. In addition, minimal orientation (six hours) and in-service training (twelve hours annually) requirements were included.

In sum, the new regulations officially moved residential care into the long-term care unit within the state regulatory system and provided much more specific guidelines for fire safety, physical environment, record keeping, and client services.

Implementation: Barriers to Effectiveness

The principal barrier to the effectiveness of SB 100 legislation has been the lack of funding to implement the changes it required. First, fiscal constraints defined the boundaries within which regulations could develop. The major impact of this constraint was on facility staffing requirements. Since the task force was charged to develop new regulations within existing industry and agency resources, many of the changes that the committees thought should be implemented, such as increased facility staffing, could not be imposed.

Thus, the regulations did not set specific qualifications for administrative staff (nor for direct care staff). "That is a real deficiency in our rules," according to one Senior Services Division (SSD) staff member, who said:

We say they [the administrators] must have knowledge, experience, or training relating to the level or kind of residents they are going to have. What we didn't do was specify the amount of training or knowledge they had to have; we don't even say they have to have a high school education . . . and in fact, we have many of them out there that who do not have a high school diploma.

As the regulations have become more complex, and the frailty of residents has increased, the need for adequately trained staff has grown even more critical to insuring quality care. As one surveyor indicated, "I rarely see a facility without medication errors in their system . . . just the basics of medical care." The Administrative Rules for Licensure for Adult Foster Homes (ORS 443.705 to 443.780) do stipulate at least annual training requirements for the licensee and resident manager, as do those rules for residential care. The provisions for foster care also allow flexibility for the division to require additional training over and above the requisite annual hours in areas found to be deficient.

In addition, the room sizes specified under the new building requirements were inadequate. Indeed, they were even less than those required by current nursing home standards. To quote one staff person:

Our rules state that the room sizes have to be 60 square feet per person. . . . In today's modern thinking, 60 square feet per person is nothing . . . it's like living in a cracker box . . . it really isn't appropriate. But we had to consider what existing facilities had in them, and many of them were just large homes or had been constructed to very minimal standards.

The passage of SB 100 slightly improved the reimbursement rate for residential care homes serving those on state assistance by adjusting the rates between the old HAs and the MED Group Care Homes. As noted earlier, group care homes had been receiving significantly greater per diem rates per resident than had residential care homes, largely because they were required to provide training and had more stringent guidelines in place. Under the new regulations, both would receive approximately $323 per month for the 1979–81 biennium if no increase was granted and $352 per month if a requested increase was approved. A staff memo concerning these figures noted that "the primary issue is one of funding.... Our required standards for these facilities [RCFs] have been and will continue to be more than present reimbursement levels."

Inadequate funding has continued to affect the ability of staff to monitor residential care facilities effectively to insure implementation of the regulations. In 1980 a single registered nurse from the Health Division was contracted to SSD to continue surveys under SSD's auspices. This nurse, along with the program coordinator from SSD, was responsible from that time until the present for all surveys of residential care facilities. The SSD staff member was also responsible for coordinating the foster home program as well as other program responsibilities within the long-term care unit. By its own admission, the staff is close to one year behind in licensing at all times. The nurse, who reviews sanitation, food services, and health services and conducts resident audits sees most facilities within a two-year period, but the program coordinator has been unable to maintain this kind of schedule for reviewing the administrative aspects of the facilities. As one surveyor notes:

Since that team member looks at specific areas such as management, building requirements, and policies and procedures, when only the nurse goes in, those parts don't get surveyed. So, some of these facilities have not had anybody looking at the administrative part of it for years . . . and while I guess the other things [physical care] are more important, the administration is the key to how the facility runs.

According to Rein (1983), adequate resources are crucial to effective administration of program mandates. Without this support, it is difficult, with even the clearest goals, to implement regulations adequately. Implementation may thus deviate considerably from the policy maker's intent. Although one might argue that any attempt to improve quality of care is better than none, one wonders what would have occurred had a more realistic proposal for funding been brought forth at the time of the passage of SB 100.

THE STATE OF RCFs UNDER SB 100: MEASURING IMPACT

Demand for RCFs

Numbers. According to the 1980 Census, 11.5 percent of the state's population was 65 years of age and older; there were 76,552 persons over the age of 75. Within the state, Multnomah County leads in numbers with 28.39 percent of households having a member 75 years of age and over.

Functional Impairment. It is very difficult to find information on households including older individuals with some impairment that limits their ability to function independently. One question from the 1980 Census asks: "Does this person have a physical, mental or other health condition which has lasted for six or more months and which limits or prevents this person from using public transportation?" Among householders 75 years of age and over, about 20 percent stated that they have a transportation disability (U.S. Bureau of the Census, Public-Use Microdata Samples, 1983). While a crude measure of functional impairment, this item at least provides an indicator of the level of functional limitation among the very elderly, that is, those most likely to consider residential care options.

State Cost Containment Strategies. The demand for residential alternatives has risen as federal and state efforts have focused on cost containment in health care for the elderly. Oregon's progressive commitment to these alternatives has definitely had an impact on the need for residential options.

In 1979 Oregon was among the first states to begin a demonstration project based on "waivers" from the Medicaid program. Under Section 2176 guidelines, the state initially requested waivers allowing for the use of more of the state's share of federal funds for in-home services, adult foster care, and other alternative services. In 1980 Oregon also received a grant from the Administration on Aging and the Health Care Financing Administration that allowed the state to study the purchase of community-based care and the effect of enhanced coordination of services in the local areas. According to a Senior Services Division Fact Sheet (2628P-s/1), the project found "that if you assess people before they enter a facility and determine they do not need that level of medical care, and place them in a community program which they desire, the state saved money and the clients were receiving quality services."

In a further effort to curb the use of costly nursing homes, in 1981 Oregon instituted a statewide system of screening all Medicaid-eligible persons before they entered a nursing home. Screening teams made recommendations as to whether individuals needed the medical services provided in a nursing home or if they could be served in a less costly and less care-intensive setting.

These early efforts and a continued commitment to cheaper, less restrictive forms of care have contributed to the demand for care options to meet the needs of elderly persons not requiring the services of a nursing home.

Supply of RCFs

Currently 103 residential care facilities, with 3,139 beds, serve the elderly in the state of Oregon.[2] The average facility has 31.2 beds, with the median-sized home having 20 resident beds. This figure is somewhat larger than the median of 14 reported by Mor et al. (1986) in their nationwide survey. This difference may reflect either the industry-wide attrition of smaller homes unable to meet the more stringent regulations in Oregon or regional differences in construction.

The design of these facilities varies considerably, with 56.4 percent of homes defined as free-standing RCFs, 29.1 percent connected to a nursing home, 9.7 percent connected to a retirement home, and 4.8 percent adjacent to both a retirement and nursing facility in a multi-level care arrangement. Interviews with state staff revealed that those RCFs attached to a nursing home or retirement home (or both) typically have better physical structures and are more likely to have licensed professional staff. As might be expected, the type of facility to which the RCF is attached also affects the level of residents in the RCF. According to one state surveyor:

> Residents in those attached to nursing homes are those that aren't quite ready for nursing care so they may be a little bit sicker.... The RCFs attached to a retirement facility have residents that are probably a little bit more ambulatory, a little more alert because they are just now coming from a place where they have been able to care for themselves.

Approximately 90 percent of the RCFs in Oregon are proprietary facilities, with the remaining 10 percent owned by nonprofit organizations such as churches and fraternal organizations. One publicly operated facility, a county home, remains in the state. Clients receiving SSI and state supplement occupy a little fewer than one-third of the existing beds in these facilities, with the remainder either private clients or vacancies. State estimates of vacancies in RCFs vary between 15 and 20 percent.

The monthly total reimbursement average for aged clients receiving state assistance in RCFs is $562.31, with $299.70 set for board and room, $220.61 for service, and $42.00 for personal needs. In Oregon the board and room rate is fixed, while the service rate varies by the capacity for which the facility is licensed; it is computed from a formula based on the factors of staffing requirements, minimum wage, other payroll expenses (OPE), and average number of residents. The present service rates were set six or seven years ago and have changed according to Consumer Price Index increases since that time. These monthly total reimbursement levels are higher than the $335 average monthly charge over all homes reported by Mor et al. (1986) and significantly higher than the $305 standard rate reported for SSI-supported clients in their study. These figures reflect an industry serving a significant number of frail older persons in Oregon and represent a sizable outlay of state and federal funds for their care. The industry, however, exhibits many problems, many of which stem from the lack of a clear policy focus and inadequate funding for the type of care expected.

Factors Affecting Supply

Interviews with state staff and private facility administrators revealed a significant list of problems facing residential care. While some of these reflect funding concerns, others grow out of a lack of common consensus on the role of residential care in the long-term care continuum. Most are interrelated.

Funding. No federal funds and extremely limited state funds exist at this time for upgrading existing facilities. This problem is particularly critical for smaller facilities serving a large proportion of public assistance clients. Continued deterioration of these facilities may lead to their closure and thus a reduction in the supply of beds for clients on public assistance.

Only one source exists for building new residential care facilities or major remodeling, and very limited state funds are available. Article XI-I (2) of the Oregon State Constitution, created by HDR 61, 1977, invested the Oregon Housing Agency (formerly the Oregon State Housing Division), with authority to sell tax-exempt, general obligation bonds to finance the Elderly/Disabled Housing Finance Program. Specifically, the program provides long-term financing (forty-year mortgages) to developers interested in building housing for those elderly and disabled whose incomes fall below the median household income for the state (currently $28,500).

The program has had a very limited impact on residential care. Since the 1977 enactment and the subsequent implementing legislation (ORS 456.515 to ORS 456.547) the program has financed the completed construction of two RCFs and sixteen congregate living facilities (Oregon Housing Agency, 1987). It is likely that limited funding for the program will continue to act as an obstacle to widespread RCF development. Interviews with loan officers of the program note that a tight bond cap has been placed on the program for the coming two years ($15 million maximum). The effect of this cap will be to reduce loans available for very large facilities. The program has targeted the remaining available funds for the development and remodeling of small (twenty beds or fewer) RCFs in the most rural areas of the state. Program staff estimate that only six to seven facilities per year will be financed under the present budget constraints.

Regulatory Environment. In addition to the limited funding available, contradictions between the regulations set forth for participation by the Housing Agency and those for licensure by the state Senior Services Division have hampered development. The existence of these contradictions provides an excellent example of the housing versus care philosophies currently at work in the residential care industry. It also illustrates what Bardach & Kagan (1982) might term a case of "regulatory unreasonableness."

Specifically, because the bonds issued are general obligation and tax-exempt, the Code of the Internal Revenue Service outlines strict requirements for how the proceeds may be used. This code specifies that bond proceeds must be used for financing "complete living units," including complete kitchen facilities with refrigerator, sink, and stove top. In order to use this source of funding for RCF construction, the units must be constructed to these specifications. These reflect the intent of the bond program to provide housing, versus a specific intent to provide care facilities.

By contrast, the administrative rules implemented through the Senior Services Division state that "all resident activities in food preparation areas shall be under the general supervision of direct care staff" (OAR 411–55–130 [10]). In other words, any cooking by residents must be done under supervision. The inclusion of this rule reflects a recognition of the frail nature of RCF residents and the care function of these facilities. The issue is further convoluted because facilities that are designated as nonprofit corporations are exempt from the Internal Revenue Service (IRS) restrictions. Therefore they do not have to include the complete cooking facilities in their construction.

This disparity has had an impact on the number of RCFs funded under the program, the costs incurred by completed projects, and the relationships among surveyors, SSD administrative staff, the Housing Agency, and providers. On the one hand, the IRS requirements have been stringently enforced by the Housing Agency. For example, a developer trying to accommodate both sets of rules might propose building a facility with only the wiring for complete kitchens, excluding the finished appliances. While lowering the cost of construction and meeting SSD requirements, this solution would not currently be accepted by the Housing Agency. In existing units built under the state program, the kitchens have been completed, but a breaker switch is located so that it is inaccessible to the residents. (In other units not financed through the state, in which stove tops were already in place, developers have gone so far as to build complete kitchen units and then wall them off. Others have merely covered the stove tops, leaving the remaining appliances). If a resident is subsequently judged too impaired to have access to the cooking unit, the power can be interrupted. Judgment of sufficient impairment is extremely subjective; measurement and monitoring of impairment levels are problematic to implement. In addition, RCF residents are becoming increasingly frail, and monitoring their fluctuating abilities over time is very difficult. With limited funds available for financing, the added costs of construction for unused kitchen facilities seem to fly in the face of reason in developing lower-cost housing for the elderly and disabled.

On the other hand, the original intent of the RCF rules regarding food preparation was to foster communal cooking activities in a safe, supervised setting. As one staff member stated, "Our [SSD] rules say that they can't use these kitchen units . . . and because of the disabilities, the frailties of the people . . . one of the reasons they are there [in the RCF] is because they can no longer handle cooking." To complicate further the implementation of the SSD rules, SSD administrative staff have supported the RCF developers in allowing construction and use of the full kitchen units, while state licensing and survey agents have held to strict enforcement of the rules.

The solution to this inconsistency remains to be found, and the inconsistency may hinder the use of the state program for residential care settings.

Administration's Commitment. Perhaps the most important factor affecting quantity and quality of residential care in the state is what staff and providers term "a lack of administrative commitment within the Department of Human Resources to RCF level care." This statement is not an unreasonable deduction on the part of staff, particularly as it relates to RCF use for clients receiving state assistance. State figures (Oregon Department of Human Resources, 1987) show a decline since 1982 for both the number of cases and the level of expenditures for residential care, in contrast to a dramatic rise both in cases and in expenditures for foster care. The reimbursement rates for service in foster care have also increased, while those in residential care have remained virtually stable for the past several years.

One explanation for this lack of commitment derives from the greater flexibility inherent in the foster care regulations. Specifically, residential care regulations (OAR 411–55–080) prohibit any resident requiring continuous nursing care. The Administrative Rules for Licensure of Adult Foster Homes (ORS 443.705 to ORS 443.780), however, allow foster homes to provide service to one person requiring nursing care at any given time. While limited to one person in each facility, this authorization has greatly enhanced the type of care allowable in foster home settings. With the number of foster care beds rising rapidly (1,422 homes with 4,600 beds as of April 1987), these nursing beds represent a significant source of long-term care.

Thus, the limitation on the level of clients allowable in residential care has reduced its usefulness, particularly for clients receiving public assistance. State administrators often report that they

feel that because they are so limited in the level of clients they can take, they are practically useless as a source of placement for our public assistance clients. It's especially true because most of the people we are placing now are either alternatives to nursing care or placements from nursing homes who no longer need that level of care, but need some nursing. RCF level has been really ignored. . . . Pleas for better payment levels are just ignored because it's not seen as a very useful level of care. And yet, there is still a need out there.

Lack of administrative commitment may not permanently deter increased funding for RCFs nor inhibit regulation reform and improvement; nor is it likely to cause the total demise of this care alternative. The absence of administrative resolve to maintain or enhance residential care has impeded improvement in the industry.

Policy Implementation: Additional Concerns

Funding and Quality Care. Not surprisingly, funding issues form the basis of many of the problems cited by all those involved in the business of residential care for older people. Funding affects not only supply, but also the quality of care. Current SSI and state supplement rates are set at levels below what staff and providers agree is adequate to provide the amount of care required by frail clients. This inadequacy has become a particularly acute problem as the level of impairment among residents has increased. While Oregon's reimbursement level is higher than the national figures reported by Mor et al. (1986), the rates are still not competitive with those charged by many of the better private facilities. The outcome, according to one staff member, is that

the homes that will take public assistance clients are the older, less attractive homes that the private person is not interested . . . and because they get most of their money from the state, it isn't adequate to do the upkeep and repairs they need to keep their buildings up... so they are in a continually deteriorating condition.... If we paid just a little more, there would be more of the private homes that would be williing to take them [Title XIX clients].

Thus, one outcome of low reimbursement rates is a two-tiered system of service provision, in which public assistance clients are housed in poorer quality facilities, while private clients can pick among a larger array of higher quality care settings. In addition, the availability of existing low-cost facilities is steadily reduced as facilities serving only low-income clients are unable to maintain facilities at the level necessary to insure licensure. State staff also admit differential levels of enforcement of provisions not related to "bed and body" care in facilities housing mostly public assistance clients. As one staff person said: "When I see how little we are paying them, I am less likely to cite deficiencies in the area of activities. In fact, we have worked very hard just to get them to provide the level of physical care required. If they are in private facilities where I know they [the providers] are getting a thousand dollars a month or better, I don't have quite that hang-up."

Inadequate funding exists for providing the number and type of surveyors needed to insure compliance and quality care in all licensed facilities. This deficiency partly derives from the inadequacy of the Keys legislation, which provided no federal support for increased monitoring and regulation at the state level. It also reflects the way in which SB 100 was engineered through the state legislature, specifically the minimization of the fiscal impact of the subsequent implementing regulations. The lag in licensing and the inadequacies in current surveys (where only one part of the survey team sees facilities regularly, and then only once every two years) are examples of critical deficiencies in the current monitoring system. A recently approved reorganization attempts to address this problem but still leaves little time for surveyors to provide what they deem necessary consultation to facilities.

A related issue is the inadequate monitoring of private-pay clients. While concerned with the rates paid for state assistance clients, almost all staff interviewed expressed even more concern for care given to private-pay clients. The Keys Amendment made no provision for oversight and sanction of facilities where no SSI recipients resided. While private facilities must be licensed and surveyed by the state, no mechanism has developed to supervise closely the care given to private-pay residents. In the state of Oregon, all Title XIX recipients are reviewed for eligibility and assessed using standardized Form 360, and their level of care is determined by a case manager who then monitors their status periodically. Thus, state assistance clients in RCFs are seen, perhaps not frequently, but at least often enough to determine if poor or inadequate care is being given.

The same case supervision is not available to those non-Title XIX (or private-pay) clients who compose the remaining two-thirds of RCF residents in the state. A surveyor's comments reflect concern for this lack of oversight:

As a person who is doing the "hands-on surveys," I think that the private-pay person is the one in the smaller, marginal facilities, although I also see the problem even in the big, newer facilities, who is on the short end of the stick. The Title XIX people are looked at by many different people—caseworkers, the screening teams sometimes—but we are limited in what we can do for private-pay people. I see a lot of low-middle-income people who can't quite qualify for assistance and yet don't have enough money to go to the really nice places. They go where they can afford to go, which is usually to a not very good situation. Those are the problem people that I have run into lately . . . the ones with decubiti, or the diabetic with severe toenail problems, etc.

Another surveyor noted:

Almost always the one that is really having problems, like a foot problem or a decubitus starting is going to be a private person . . . there just isn't anybody coming in and looking at them very regularly. So, they don't get the care that the public assistance clients do, and that's ironic because they are often paying twice as much or more for their care. I think the providers try to keep them longer than they should, and we really don't have the staff to monitor them.

Quality of Caregivers. While state staff are concerned with issues related to funding levels, they also focus on the characteristics of those administering and providing direct care to RCF residents. While the lack of adequate reimbursement contributes to an inability to provide quality care to public assistance clients, the most commonly cited problems, beyond financing, are poorly trained staff and high staff turnover. Direct-care staff show the most fluctuation, with most personal aide positions in RCFs offering only minimum wage or slightly above for demanding work with an increasingly frail and sick population. In addition, most staff are poorly trained. The administrator may have few resources for teaching and training a constantly changing group of aides. These problems are similar to those cited by Mor et al. (1986) that exist in residential homes nationwide. As one Oregon surveyor noted, "The requirements for the administrator are so minimal that usually they don't have the insight or know-how to provide inservice for their staff . . . so their own lack of training is often the source of the problem."

While state staff and providers also acknowledge the problems associated with meeting the various state regulations and dealing with surveyors from multiple agencies, most felt the issues of adequate funding, staff, and training were far more critical. One administrator commented that if these issues could be addressed, the need for extensive regulation and monitoring would be reduced. The lesser importance given to the surveyor's role as a barrier to providers differs from that cited by the provider respondents in the national survey by Mor et al. (1986). Since no complete survey of providers in Oregon was undertaken for this study, this finding may be viewed with caution. It may reflect only the opinions of the providers and state staff interviewed.

State staff also recognize the need for increased consultation with providers.

This need reflects a role for regulators that Bardach and Kagan (1982) have termed "the good inspector." While some state staff feel that residential care does not receive enough oversight, surveyors themselves expressed the desire to act more as consultants and problem solvers, working with the administrators rather than focusing on their "policie" function. As Bardach and Kagan noted, this desire reflects a recognition by regulatory agencies that when violations and deficiencies occur as a result of "employee inattentiveness, inadequate supervision, corporate misperception of risks, or ignorance of preventive measures" (p. 143) the regulatory agency may be able to teach the regulated enterprise. This approach would ideally foster better relationships and minimize recurrences of violations. A state surveyor expressed this desire:

I'd love to be able to go in and say to a provider . . . "I'm in the area today, do you have any problems you would like me to work on with you?" I think I have gained the confidence of quite a number of them to do that. . . . On the other hand, on the state's side, if people are going to go into this business, they better know what they are doing . . . why should we fund a lot of consultation?

Compounding the training problem is the constant turnover of administrators. One surveyor noted that new administrators are often unaware of the meaning of the rules and regulations. When asked if administrators should also be expected to understand a little of the nature of care for older clients, including some knowledge of the impact of various chronic illnesses, state staff responded that they were willing to settle for administrators who possessed a basic understanding of the expectations inherent in the regulations.

Medical Nature of RCFs. The growing "medicalization" of residential care facilities is also of concern to state staff. As one respondent succinctly stated:

It has always been kind of a gray line to know whether they are residential care or ICF [intermediate care], and it's getting grayer as the days pass on. Particularly, with the pressure to move people out of nursing homes, we see people in RCFs who need a lot more custodial care.

In a related discussion, one respondent noted the increasing use of intermittent nursing care in RCFs. For example, a home health professional may come in to administer daily injections, change sterile dressings, or provide other services that are temporary or short-term in nature. These types of services have generally been acceptable under the current regulations. State staff noted that in the last few years surveyors have become increasingly generous in allowing this type of nursing care. There is growing pressure from those in the industry and even from some state representatives to "break down the barriers between nursing homes and residential care facilities." Caution, however, was urged. "I think we have to be really, really cautious. . . . It's a pretty fine line and if we start breaking down that barrier even more [between levels of care] and openly permitting some heavier care in RCFs, I think we are going to get lots of flak from the nursing home industry . . . and rightly so. They have to meet different regulations, especially in terms of staffing . . . and we have problems enough now with foster homes where we have people of all levels of care and some receiving pretty heavy care."

The evidence then clearly indicates a trend, evident in both foster homes and residential care facilities, to provide expanded medical services to aged residents. Yet the regulations were designed for facilities seen primarily as protective housing for those individuals needing some supervision and basic assistance with personal care. Current facility staff is too limited in numbers and inadequately trained to provide more intensive medical care services. Moreover, state staff acknowledge their own inability to monitor closely those facilities that may provide care beyond the level for which they are licensed. One surveyor noted that "there are also some retirement homes that are starting to provide care, and if we really are serious about licensing all of those that provide care, we should be beating the bushes to see that they are licensed." As the level of impairment rises throughout the housing and care continuum, facilities will try to meet the needs of elderly clients, regardless of their physical or mental decline, in order to maintain occupancy in an increasingly competitive market.

One additional trend adds to the "medicalization" syndrome. Staff at all levels of the state pointed to the increase in requests for residential care licensure by nursing homes and by retirement homes wishing to add nursing care units. The scenario proceeds as follows. The nursing or retirement home adds beds designated as RCF level of care. In retirement homes, most typically, they construct a new wing, designed and built to nursing home specifications, but they call the beds RCF for original licensure. In existing nursing facilities, they may build an addition or merely activate beds as available. Then, as the Certificate of Need Process allows them a 10 percent increase in ICF/SNF beds every two years or as they eventually get CON approval, they funnel those RCF beds into their ICF level of designation. This backdoor technique to get around the CON process also contributes to an increasing number of medically oriented residential care units, both in structural design and philosophy of care. (This practice may be limited by the OBRA (1987) legislation deleting ICF-level care.)

With all the evidence available regarding the changing needs of the residential care population, the state has undertaken some efforts at reform. It is, however, important to bear in mind the caution given earlier by a state surveyor. The state is in the curious position of acknowledging and trying to address the increasingly medical nature of residential care facilities, while avoiding encroachment on the care functions of the nursing home industry. Recent trends suggest that the housing versus care dilemma has come closer to a resolution, perhaps unacknowledged, by those regulating and monitoring residential care facilities. That is, there is some recognition of the level of medical care now being provided in these facilities, and there is a sense of responsibility for insuring that the care given is of a high quality. This trend is most clearly seen in the three levels of care now designated within adult foster care.[3] The outcome is that residential care has been formally included in the long-term care system of the state.

As we conclude this review of Oregon's experience in developing and implementing policy related to residential care, it is important to recognize the progress that has been made. Oregon, with passage of SB 100, made substantial progress toward the goal of improving licensing and standards for residential care just prior to the passage of the Keys Amendment in 1977. Indeed, the drafting of new administrative rules had begun that fall, and Oregon seemed a step ahead from that time forth. Significant advances have been made in fire safety and medical supervision. Yet the problems of coping with an increasingly frail client group with limited state resources still exist.

More importantly, the impression of the increasing impairment levels of residents is largely anecdotal on the part of those at the state level involved in developing policy and drafting regulations for implementation. No quantitative data adequately evaluate the level of impairment in this population; similarly, no information exists on the types of services needed by these residents. Discussion regarding the suitability of providing these services within the RCF setting is limited. This type of data would ideally form the basis for policy changes directed at meeting the service needs of the RCF population.

One source of better data may emerge as a result of recent changes in Oregon's monitoring of RCFs. A significant outcome of recent changes is broader implementation of RCF resident assessments, including evaluation and assessment of private-pay residents. Previously, only those residents screened for Title XIX eligibility were evaluated, using the state Form 360, a multi-item, comprehensive functional assessment instrument. Following organizational changes, all Title XIX clients will continue to be evaluated, as will a specific percentage of all residents in each licensed facility. The schedule for administering Form 360 provides for interviews of (1) all residents in facilities of six to twenty-four beds, (2) fifty percent of residents in facilities of twenty-five to forty-nine beds, and (3) twenty-five percent of residents in homes of more than fifty beds. A small random sample of private-pay residents will therefore be reviewed at least every two years.

Some state staff seriously question the adequacy of Form 360 for providing the type and amount of information needed to monitor the increasingly frail residents. In addition, while the infrequent evaluations cannot adequately monitor care in specific cases over time, the provision allows for some oversight of private-pay residents. The inclusion of all residents in the assessment process also signals a recognition of the gap cited by state staff. The data collected will begin to address the dearth of information currently available on the health and functional status of older persons residing in residential care facilities.

While broader use of Form 360 may contribute to limited improvements in understanding current RCF users, further attention must be given to determining the characteristics of residential care users and the types and levels of services needed to provide for their care. The following chapter provides an example of the type of research that seems critical to a more definitive federal and state policy regarding the role of residential care. Examination of the characteristics of residential care consumers should provide insight into the care needs of this population and illuminate many of the issues raised here. Until an accurate picture of those elderly persons who reside in these settings is obtained, current policy and planning will be less than effective in insuring the quality of their care. At least on the surface, the housing versus care dilemma will remain.

NOTES

1. To increase participation, anonymity was guaranteed to all state staff members who participated in interviews. Therefore, only general acknowledgements are given with quotes in this chapter.

2. Facility characteristics are current as of April 1, 1987. Reimbursement levels are from rate schedules effective January 1, 1987, and current through July 1987.

3. ORS 443.705 to 443.825, Administrative Rules for Licensure of Adult Foster Homes, State of Oregon, became effective November 1, 1988. These rules classify adult foster homes as Class I, Class II, or Class III based upon the qualifications of the provider or resident manager of the home and the type of care provided residents. ORS 411–50–443 defines the care levels as follows: "(2) A provider with a Class I license may only admit residents who need assistance in up to four activities of daily living (ADLs). No nursing tasks may be delegated except for routine maintenance of oral medications. The resident must be in stable condition." Class II providers "may provide care for residents who require assistance in all activities of daily living, but are not dependent in more than three activities of daily living. Routine nursing tasks may be delegated to the provider and qualified staff under the Board of Nursing Rules." Finally, a provider with a Class III designation "may provide care for residents who are dependent in activities of daily living, except that no more than one bed-care or totally dependent person may be in residence at one time. Complex tasks will be performed by a registered nurse or may be delegated under the Board of Nursing Rules, with written justification by both physician and registered nurse and specific approval granted by the Division."

CHAPTER 6

Characteristics of Residential Care Facility Residents: An Exploratory Analysis

The demand for residential care services in recent decades has spurred tremendous growth in these care alternatives, yet little is known about the older persons who reside in these settings. That is, scant attention has been paid to discerning the types and levels of their impairment. Current regulations and types of care provided evolve without this critical information.

In general, the available literature describes the population as similar to that of nursing homes. The residents tend to be older than the general elderly segment of the population and more likely to be female. These factors alone do not indicate the types of impairment in this population or provide insight into the service needs of these individuals. Only the recent article by Mor et al. (1986) has attempted to assess more clearly the characteristics and needs of this population.

This chapter analyzes research conducted in one residential care facility in an attempt to describe in greater detail the characteristics and care needs of this population. The research reported here is not meant to be a definitive analysis of residential care. Nor does it provide the depth of analysis needed to compare residential populations across the states. It was undertaken as an exploratory analysis and is useful as an example of the types of research that are needed in this field.

CONCEPTUALIZATION

In the literature on the variety of long-term care services, surprisingly few articles are available. Of these, a dozen or so dealt with the variables associated with the decision to place an older person in a nursing home; many were anecdotal. From these studies it is possible to identify some basic factors that distinguish those individuals who enter the long-term care system via the various levels of housing and care options.

In a seminal article, Dick, Friedsam, and Martin (1964) described research exploring the factors associated with nursing home placement. Specifically, they examined the residential patterns of aged persons prior to institutionalization and found that the decision to enter an institution was related to changes in health, changes in the family structure, and gender. Thus, early research suggested that the decision was not based on one variable alone, but that a combination of demographic, social, psychological, and financial factors identified those older persons likely to enter a nursing home. Saul (1969), in a study of blind applicants to one nursing home, found that the absence of a caring person and the opportunity to continue roles and relationships were critical factors in decision making. Brody (1969) noted that the attitude toward institutionalization, both on the part of the applicants and their families, as well as the number of physical problems present, discriminated applicants to a voluntary home from nonapplicants. Looking at a broader population and attempting to develop professional assessment instruments to identify elderly persons with a high risk of institutional placement, Sherwood, Morris, and Barnhart (1975) listed the factors of social isolation, lack of social services, and loss of support from family and friends, as well as financial, physical, and mental status. Although Townsend (1963), in a review of the nursing home residents of England and Wales, noted essentially the same key variables, Sherwood, Morris, and Barnhart (1975) stressed the interaction between variables, specifically the effect of impairment in more than one area as causal factors.

Additional evidence has suggested the importance of living arrangements, marital status, availability of social supports, financial situation, gender, race, and education, as well as physical and mental status, in determining who is at risk for long-term care (Townsend, 1963, 1965; Davis & Gibbin, 1971; Barney, 1973; Palmore, 1976; Vicente, Wiley, & Carrington, 1979; Greenberg & Ginn, 1979; Anderson, Patten, & Greenberg, 1980; Butler & Newacheck, 1981). The variables chosen for analysis in this research reflect the multidimensional factors associated with the use of long-term care services—in other words, those variables most likely to discriminate residential care consumers from the larger elderly population.

QUESTIONS ADDRESSED BY THE STUDY

The exploratory analysis undertaken was designed to address specific questions regarding the residential care population. Specifically, the hypotheses were generated from the following general questions:

1. What are the demographic characteristics of the residential care population?
2. Is the residential care population significantly more frail than older persons currently using other housing and care options in the community?

3. In which functional areas are the residential care consumers significantly more frail (or showing more impairment) than their counterparts in less restrictive community care settings?
4. How do these levels of impairment relate to current policy and regulation in the field of residential care?

HYPOTHESES

Based on previous research on the characteristics of elderly persons using other types of long-term care services (that is, nursing homes and day care), anecdotal evidence from providers, and my own experience, I developed the following hypotheses regarding the characteristics of those elderly persons residing in residential care facilities. I predicted that RCF residents would

1. show greater levels of mental impairment than the alternative community sample;
2. show greater levels of impairment in the instrumental activities of daily living than the alternative community sample;
3. show greater levels of impairment in the physical activities of daily living than the alternative community sample;
4. show greater levels of impairment in affect functioning than the alternative community sample;
5. rate their well-being in the areas of physical and mental health lower than would those respondents in less restrictive housing/care settings; and
6. report a less effective social support system than those respondents in the alternative community sample.

METHODOLOGY

To address the research questions posed, a study was undertaken of the characteristics of residents in a private new residential care facility in the Northwest, and a sample was drawn from the population of this facility. A standardized comprehensive functional assessment instrument was administered to twenty-five residents, three times each, at three-month intervals during a six-month period. Social, demographic, and functional status information was obtained on this sample of residents beginning with their application and move to the facility. Each resident was then interviewed again with the same protocol at three months following admission and at six months following admission. In addition, site-specific data were collected from the facility files regarding medical diagnoses at the time of admission and the type and intensity of services provided to the residents by the facility (that is, the care plan) throughout the study period.

To address the question of how these residents differ from older persons living in other housing settings, a community sample of twenty-five persons was also administered the assessment, using the same repeated measures.

Sample

The residential care sample was chosen from applicants to a new residential care facility; it was limited to those who made application between January 1985 and January 1986. A convenience sample was used, based on the applicant's willingness to participate and ability to self-report. In this instance, convenience also indicates that, at random, applicants submitted to an assessment using the Geriatric Assessment Testing and Evaluation System (GATES)[1] instrument and gave permission to participate in the remaining two interviews. It does not mean that every nth applicant was chosen. Rather, as in much policy and applied research, it means that a staff person was available to do the assessment, and the applicant met the above criteria. This process continued until a sample of twenty-five was obtained. (Oversampling was done to insure an end-study of twenty-five). This sample was administered the GATES instrument three times during a six-month period (at three-month intervals). Both the resident sample and the community sample were informed of their rights as subjects and asked to sign the informed consent form. During this same time frame a community comparison sample of twenty-five individuals was also chosen. This sample was obtained by using the facility's marketing records to contact individuals who had expressed interest in the RCF chosen for this study (that is, they had come for a tour, called for information, or made application but moved elsewhere). On contact, they were questioned regarding their willingness to participate. This community sample therefore includes those individuals who for some reason were searching for housing with some services provided but subsequently made a housing/care choice other than residential care. At the time of the first interview, respondents in the comparison sample were living in the following settings: own home (nine); private apartment (three); with adult children (one); retirement apartment (eight); adult foster care (two); and nursing home (two). The comparison sample was also administered the GATES instrument plus additional questions three times during a six-month period. The subjects were all at least 65 years of age, had made at least one contact with the RCF, and were capable of self-report.

Several issues must be addressed regarding the sample chosen for this research. First, as in most field research, obtaining a true random sample was not feasible, and the sample size is small. Time and staff constraints, as well as facility policies, allowed for neither true randomization nor large sample size. One of the assumptions of analysis of variance (as well as other multivariate techniques) is normal distribution, which is more likely with large sample sizes and random assignment. The violation of this assumption can affect the F-test outcomes. While some literature shows that F-tests are not adversely affected by deviations from normality (that is, they are robust), extreme deviations would affect the levels of significance.

Second, limiting the sample to those capable of self-report limits generalization to the residential care population as a whole. Anecdotal evidence suggests that residential care may be the first alternative for those older persons exhibiting noticeable impairment in mental function. Preliminary evidence reported here suggests that even those selected for this study show significantly more impairment than the community sample. Unfortunately, observational assessment instruments for measuring functional status in those persons incapable of self-report could not be located. It is of interest to note that the developers of the GATES instrument originally designed another version of it for use with the mentally impaired. Their instrument was to be completed by an informant close to the older person. In the initial testing of both instruments, both self-report and informant, the informant instrument was found to be unreliable as a measure of the person's functional status and was abandoned.

The residential care sample also represents a particular income level. With private monthly rates approaching those of nursing home care, only a small sector of older persons was likely to choose the residence. It was assumed, however, that the impairments that brought them to the RCF setting were similar to those that would compel those with less income to choose less costly RCF alternatives.

The demographic comparison between the samples shown in Table 6.1 indicates no significant difference between them except in age. RCF residents tended to be older.

Data Collection

Conduct of Interviews. Data were collected in personal interviews with all RCF residents in the sample. The assessment was designed to be administered as part of the application process. Follow-up interviews were conducted at the residents' convenience, most often in their own rooms in the RCF. Interviews with the community sample were arranged by the interviewer. The initial interview was always in person, most often in the residence of the respondent. Subsequent interviews were conducted in person if possible, but one interview at both time 1 and time 2 was conducted by phone to insure continued participation by the subject.

All interviewers were professional staff and included social worker (MSW), an MSW social work student, a gerontology specialist in the field of activities, and the Social Services director of the facility. Each interviewer was trained in the use of the instrument, using the training package provided by its developers. Bimonthly briefings were held to review issues concerning the instrument, respondent concerns, and scheduling of follow-up interviews.

Instrument. For this research, an existing comprehensive functional assessment instrument, which addressed the variables of interest based on previous theoretical work and on the author's experience, was chosen to develop a profile of residential care consumers. The instrument chosen was the Geriatric Assessment Testing and Evaluation System (GATES) Comprehensive Assessment Form de-

Table 6.1
Demographic Analysis of Respondents

Variable	RCF (N=25)		Community (N=25)		Total (N=50)		t results
Age	X̄=83.84		X̄=77.28				<.001
	n	%	n	%	n	%	
Gender							
Male	6	24	4	16	10	20	NS
Female	19	76	21	84	40	80	
Marital Status							
Married	8	32	6	24	14	28	NS
Single	-	-	2	8	2	4	
Widowed	16	64	16	64	32	64	
Divorced/Separated	1	4	1	4	2	4	
Ethnicity							
Caucasian	25	100	24	96	49	98	NS
Black	-		1	4	1	2	
Education							
0-4 Years	1	4	-	-	1	2	NS
5-8 Years	3	12	2	8	5	10	
Incomplete HS	5	20	5	20	10	20	
High School Grad.	2	8	3	12	5	10	
Post HS -Bus/Trade	2	8	1	4	3	6	
1-3 Years College	6	24	9	36	15	30	
College Grad.	4	16	2	8	6	12	
Post Graduate	2	8	3	12	5	10	
Income							
$20,000 +	14	56	7	28	21	42	NS
$10-20,000	9	36	12	48	21	42	
$5-10,000	-	-	5	20	5	10	
Not Reported	2	8	1	4	3	6	

Note: Demographic data reflect status of respondents at the time of first interview.

veloped by Cairl, Pfeiffer, and Keller (undated) of the Suncoast Gerontology Center.

While a large number of functional assessment instruments have been developed (Kane & Kane, 1981; Israel et al., 1984), many were not designed for specific research purposes and are not applicable in all settings. From a review of assessment instruments conducted by this author (Petersen & Baggett, 1985), the GATES was chosen. This instrument provides for a comprehensive analysis of elderly functional status, in a form judged to be effective in the interview process (ease of administration, flow, little resistance on part of respondents, length). It was also the instrument chosen by the participating RCF for an intake and assessment tool. In addition, some testing of the instrument had been completed; communication with the instrument's developers was established.

The GATES Comprehensive Assessment Form measures numerous domains and subdomains of functioning, providing subdomain scores that can be examined in their original form or used to establish a risk score for the individual. The domains and subdomains addressed include:

1. Demographics
2. Social Resources
    A. Family and social supports
    B. Satisfaction with family and social supports
    C. Activities
3. Mental Health
    A. Cognitive
    B. Affective
    C. Subjective well-being—mental health
    D. Mental health service utilization
    E. Mental health perceived needs
4. Physical Health
    A. Health status
    B. Medications
    C. Health habits
    D. Nutrition
    E. Physical health service utilization
    F. Physical health perceived needs
    G. Subjective well-being—physical health
5. Special Equipment
6. ADL (Activities of Daily Living)
    A. Instrumental ADL
    B. Physical ADL

While data were collected on all subdomains, many of which will be used in the descriptive analysis, only those subdomain scores used for the analysis of variance (those variables included in the research hypotheses) will be described in operational terms below.

Additional questions were of interest to this author and were included as an addendum to the standardized instrument. These included information concerning the respondents' housing history, service use history, and method by which each respondent had first learned of the residential care facility. Individuals in the community sample were also asked to describe the decision-making process involved in choosing their current housing.

Operationalization of Variables. Only those variables that are posed in the hypotheses and that are the subject of the analysis reported in this study are presented here.

1. Mental health/cognitive status: GATES incorporates the standardized Short Portable Mental Status Questionnaire [SPMSQ] (Pfeiffer, 1975) to assess current mental status. Designed specifically for use with the elderly, the SPMSQ consists of ten items directed toward testing several aspects of intellectual functioning, including short-term memory, long-term memory, orientation to surroundings, information about current events, and the capacity to perform serial mathematical tasks. A total scale score is obtained by summing the error responses and adjusting for education.

2. Subjective well-being/mental health: Three items address the older respondents' subjective mental well-being. These include: (a) All in all, how much happiness would you say you find in life today? (b) On the whole, how satisfied would you say you are with your way of life today? and (c) Is your mental health or emotional health now better, about the same, or worse than it was five years ago? A sum from the three items, using their weighted response codes, forms the overall subdomain score.

3. Mental health/affect: GATES incorporates the standardized Short Psychiatric Evaluation Schedule [SPES] (Pfeiffer, 1979) to address the affective component of mental health. Specifically, SPES consists of fifteen items for identifying functional psychiatric disorder, including depression.

4. Subjective well-being/physical health: A three-item subdomain addresses the respondents' subjective physical well-being. Items include: (a) How would you rate your overall health at the present time—excellent, good, fair, or poor? (b) Is your health now better, about the same, or worse than it was five years ago? and (c) How much do your health troubles stand in the way of your doing the things you want to do—not at all, a little (some), or a great deal? A total scale score is obtained by summing indicated items.

5. Instrumental activities of daily living (IADL): A six-item subdomain addresses the individual's ability to perform common instrumental activities of daily living. Specifically the items ask respondents to report whether they can perform the functions without help or with some help or whether they are unable to perform the task at all. Tasks include using the telephone, shopping for groceries or clothes, preparing meals, doing housework, taking medications, and handling their own money. A total subdomain score is obtained by summing scores for each item.

6. Physical activities of daily living: A six-item subdomain addresses the individual's ability to perform common physical activities of daily living. As with the IADLs, five of the items ask respondents to report whether they can perform the functions without help or with some help or whether they are unable

Figure 6.1
Two-Way Analysis of Variance with Repeated Measures Design

FACTOR 2	Time 1	Time 2	Time 3
Housing Type A (RCF)	25	25	25
Housing Type B (Other)	25	25	25

to perform the task at all. Tasks including eating, dressing and undressing self, caring for their own appearance, walking, and bathing or showering. A sixth item elicits information regarding continence and asks respondents whether they never, occasionally, frequently, or always have trouble getting to the bathroom on time.

7. Social resources—family and social supports: A seven-item subdomain of the GATES addresses the availability of family and social resources. Items include (a) marital status and ability of spouse, if applicable, to care for self; (b) current living arrangement (who lives with respondent); (c) major helper; (d) currently surviving children; (e) visits by children; (f) frequency of telephone visits; (g) frequency of in-person visits with others.

Methods of Analysis

All descriptive and multivariate analyses of the data were completed using the CRUNCH Statistical Package. For purposes of description, the frequency function was used to produce standard frequency tables, and the t-test function was used to examine differences in the descriptive analysis between the two groups.

A two-way analysis of variance with repeated measures was used to examine changes within the groups over time and between groups on the variables chosen, based on previous theoretical evidence. A visual representation of the study design and analysis of variance is shown in Figure 6.1.

Specifically, a two-way analysis of covariance for a factorial design with equal cell frequencies (twenty-five in each) was used to examine the effects of the two variables, time and place of residence, on the individual and group scores obtained using GATES. In other words, mean scores on the various subscales within GATES that were chosen for this analysis could be compared across place of residence and over time. The covariate, age, was shown to be a factor significantly different between the two groups in the demographic analysis and thus was added to the model to control for differences in the dependent variables that might be a function of age.

Table 6.2
Length of Residence in Metropolitan Study Area

Length	RCF (N=25) n	RCF (N=25) %	Community (N=25) n	Community (N=25) %	Total (N=50) n	Total (N=50) %
Less than 6 months	8	32	2	8	10	20
6 months - one year	2	8	4	16	6	12
1 - 5 years	1	4	2	8	3	6
6 - 10 years	2	8	3	12	5	10
11-15 years	1	4	1	4	2	4
20 years or more	11	44	13	52	24	48

DESCRIPTIVE ANALYSIS

At the time of the first interview the two groups differed significantly in age, with a mean age of 83 years in the RCF sample and 77 years in the community sample. Both samples were predominantly white, female, and widowed, with annual incomes above $10,000; approximately half of both groups had attended college for some period of time. This finding is not surprising. The RCF under study was located in a suburban area of a large Northwest city and was built for and marketed primarily for an upper-middle-income population. In addition, with rates approaching those of nursing home care (varying from $1,049 to $2,400 per month), only a select portion of the population would consider the facility an option or be accepted for admission. The descriptive information to follow represents the samples at the time of the first interview, except where noted.

Information was collected regarding the previous residence of both samples and the length of time they had resided in the metropolitan area. As shown in Table 6.2, 40 percent of those in the RCF group had lived in the area for less than one year. This evidence, along with that provided by facility records, reflects the trend by adult children to move their frail parents closer to their own residence. Several of the respondents had moved to the facility from the East Coast and the Midwest in order to be near their children. Still, approximately half of both samples had resided in the area for twenty years or more.

In addition, more of the community sample than the RCF group were either currently residing in their own homes or had resided in their own homes prior to the study (that is, many of the individuals in this sample moved to another type of housing/care alternative as a result of the search during which they examined the RCF under study). In general, Table 6.3 reveals that more of the elderly persons in the RCF group had lived in other sheltered settings, including five who had lived in either a private home or apartment in a retirement community and six who had resided in a foster care home or nursing home immediately prior to the study period.

The remainder of this descriptive analysis focuses on the variables that were thought most likely to reflect differences in the level of frailty between the two

Table 6.3
Previous Location

Length	RCF (N=25) n	RCF (N=25) %	Community (N=25) n	Community (N=25) %	Total (N=50) n	Total (N=50) %
Own home in community	5	20	8	32	18	36
Child's home	1	4	1	4	2	4
Apartment	7	28	3	12	13	26
Retirement community(Home)	3	12	1	4	4	8
Retirement home	2	8	8	32	3	6
Foster care home	3	12	2	8	3	6
Nursing home	3	12	2	8	4	8
Other	1	4	-	-	3	6

Note: Previous location refers to the respondents' location immediately prior to the first interview. For the RCF sample this refers to their living situation prior to their move to the RCF.

Table 6.4
Health Indicators (Frequencies)

Indicators	RCF (N=25) n	RCF (N=25) %	Community (N=25) n	Community (N=25) %	Total (N=50) n	Total (N=50) %	t results
Total # of Illnesses (Self-Report)							
1-3	7	28	10	40	17	34	NS
4-6	14	56	12	48	26	52	
7-9	4	16	3	12	7	14	
Mean	4.80		4.32				
Total # of Medications (Self-Report for Comnuity, facility records for RCF)							
0-2	7	28	13	52	20	40	<0.05
3-5	8	32	10	40	18	36	
6-8	5	20	2	8	7	14	
9 or more	5	20	-	-	5	10	
Mean	5.64		2.67				

groups. These variables primarily relate to physical health. Two variables, self-reported illness and total number of medications, were chosen as physical health indicators. The results are presented in Table 6.4. The evidence indicates a significant difference in medication use between the two groups, with the RCF population averaging a greater number of medications. The number of reported illnesses between the two groups shows no significant difference. Some caution, however, is needed with reference to medications. The RCF data were collected

Table 6.5
Respondents' Ability to Take Own Medications (Self-Report)

Ability	RCF (N=25)		Community (N=25)		Total (N=50)		t results
	n	%	n	%	n	%	
Without help	13	52	23	92	36	72	<0.01
With some help	12	48	2	8	14	28	
Unable to perform	-	-	-	-	-	-	

Table 6.6
Health Care Utilization by Respondents During Six Months Prior to Initial Interview

Variable	RCF (N=25)		Community (N=25)		Total (N=50)		t results
	n	%	n	%	n	%	
# of Times Seen by Physician							
0-5	21	84	21	84	42	84	NS
6-8	2	8	1	4	3	6	
9 or more	2	8	3	12	5	10	
Days of Illness[a]							
0-10	24	96	24	96	48	96	NS
11-20	-	-	1	4	1	2	
21 or more	1	4	-	-	1	2	
Hospital Stays							
0-1	20	80	24	96	44	88	NS
2	5	20	1	4	6	12	
3 or more	-	-	-	-	-	-	

[a]Category does not include days in a hospital or nursing home.

from facility records. By Oregon law, medication orders must also include nonprescription medicines. While the community respondents were encouraged to include nonprescription drugs in their own self-reported count, evidence from other research suggests that use of nonprescription medication is often underreported. When Table 6.4 is viewed in conjunction with Table 6.5, it becomes evident that, compared to community respondents, residents of the RCF not only take a greater number of medications, but also report that they need some help in taking their medication.

Three descriptive variables were also chosen to represent health care utilization by the two samples; the results appear in Table 6.6. The two groups showed little difference in their visits to physicians, days of illness, or number of hospital

Table 6.7
Respondents Reporting Adherence to a Special Diet

Special Diet	RCF (N=25)		Community (N=25)		Total (N=50)		t results
	n	%	n	%	n	%	
Yes	7	28	5	20	12	24	NS
No	18	72	20	80	38	76	

Table 6.8
Respondents' Reported Levels of Incontinence[a]

Incontinence	RCF (N=25)		Community (N=25)		Total (N=50)		t results
	n	%	n	%	n	%	
No	13	52	21	84	34	68	NS
Occasionally	12	48	3	12	15	30	
Frequently	-	-	-	-	-	-	
Always[b]	-	-	1	4	1	2	

[a]Question asks, "Do you ever have trouble getting to the bathroom on time?"
[b]"Always" denotes presence of catheter or colostomy.

stays in the six months prior to their initial interview. These findings closely reflect those of Mor et al. (1986). While the two studies are not directly comparable, a slightly lower percentage (9.8) of their total sample had been in the hospital two or more times in the past year. In the present study, 12 percent reported having been hospitalized twice in the past six months. In days of illness and physician visits, the two analyses suggest a similar pattern of health care utilization.

Anecdotal evidence suggests that, in addition to moving to a sheltered setting for the monitoring of medications, some older persons move to a sheltered setting in order to cope with special diet needs when they can no longer provide for their own meals. Therefore the numbers of respondents requiring a special dietary regimen were also examined. As shown in Table 6.7, no statistically significant difference was found between the RCF sample and the community group.

In addition, continence of bowel and bladder has been viewed as a critical determinant for sheltered care placement. In this instance, incontinence has been cited as a barrier to placing some individuals since facilities or homes have denied access to residents requiring this level of care. The RCF under study had such an admission criterion. The applicants were required at the time of application to report continence levels. If they currently used some support (for example, adult absorbent pads), then they needed to show that they were able to use these supportive devices without assistance. In addition, they had to show that they did not require help in getting to and from the toilet. Table 6.8 presents

Table 6.9
Types of Assistance Provided to RCF Residents (N = 25)

	Time 1		Time 2		Time 3	
Type of Assistance	n	%	n	%	n	%
Vital signs monthly	6	24	13	52	12	48
Vital signs > monthly	3	12	10	40	12	48
Shower assistance	18	72	16	64	16	64
Dressing assist, partial	3	12	5	20	5	20
Dressing assist, total	2	8	2	8	3	12
Oral care	1	4	2	8	2	8
Nail care	4	16	9	36	11	44
Escort to meals	3	12	1	4	2	8
Continence care	-	-	2	8	3	12
Eating assistance	1	4	1	4	1	4
Bowel/bladder training	1	4	1	4	2	8
Remind of ADl's	1	4	-	-	-	-
Remind of meals/activities	8	32	7	28	6	24
Walk/range of motion assist	3	12	1	4	3	12
Orientation	2	8	-	-	-	-
Apartment safety check	1	4	1	4	1	4
Apartment clean 1 x wk	1	4	1	4	1	4
Extra nutritional care	1	4	2	8	3	12
Assist with devices	1	4	3	12	3	12
Additional medical assist	4	16	8	32	9	36
Skin care	2	8	3	12	3	12
Mean # Areas Given Assistance[a]	$\bar{X}=2.64$		$\bar{X}=6.60$		$\bar{X}=3.90$	

Note: Numbers in table reflect multiple areas of assistance given each respondent.

data on continence, with the RCF sample exhibiting no statistically significant difference on this variable compared to community respondents. The admission rule would predict this outcome. Of interest, however, is the fact that at time 3, the RCF sample did show an increase in the number of responses in the categories "frequently" and "always"; t-tests between the two samples at time 3 report a p result significant at the .05 level. This change, with the RCF population exhibiting greater difficulty with continence after admission, has policy implications for care that will be discussed later.

Descriptive Analysis: Focus on RCF Residents

To identify more clearly the characteristics of the RCF population, additional data were collected from facility records regarding sample residents. First, upon admission, residents were determined to need one of two levels of care, with the upper level of care denoting additional services to be provided to the resident. Table 6.9 presents data regarding the types of assistance provided to residents at both levels. The range of assistance is broad and indicates the areas of greatest impairment among the residents. For example, over two-thirds needed assistance

Table 6.10
Primary Diagnoses of RCF Respondents (N = 25)

Diagnosis	n	%
Alzheimer's/other dementia	5	20
Anemia	3	12
Arteriosclerosis	3	12
Arthritis/Rheumatism	11	44
Bowel impairment	2	8
Cancer	3	12
Cataracts	4	16
Circulation impairment	3	12
Depression	9	36
Diabetes	2	8
Endocrine system impairments	6	24
Fractures/effects of	4	16
Glaucoma	1	4
Gynecological impairment	2	8
Heart disease	8	32
High blood pressure	10	40
Liver disease	2	8
Neurological other/epilepsy, seizure	1	4
Obesity	1	4
Osteoporosis	4	16
Parkinson's disease	3	12
Psychiatric disorder	1	1
Respiratory disease	2	8
Skin disorders	5	20
Stomach disorders	6	24
Stroke/effects of	3	12
Urinary tract disorder	7	28

Note: Numbers reflect multiple diagnoses per resident.

with shower/bath, and one-third needed to be reminded of meals and other activities. By time 2, almost one-half needed to have their vital signs taken more than once per month, and another one-third needed partial or total assistance with dressing.

The change in the amount of assistance over time appears to indicate that the RCF population is a frail, older group, with fluctuating physical and mental status. The curvilinear relationship in Table 6.9 may also indicate that, at time 2, residents were requiring more assistance as a result of post-move trauma. That is, the first three months of residence in a facility may cause stress upon an individual, who then requires more assistance than at time 1. While the individuals in the sample chosen for this study might also be seen as the "most capable" of the facility population (because of the requirements for study participation), they still required assistance with numerous activities of daily living and medical supervision. Table 6.10 presents the primary diagnoses of RCF respondents. Each respondent had multiple diagnoses, with a mean of 4.96 per resident and a median of 5. The high incidence of depression among the sample is of interest. While RCFs may provide medical care for common disorders such

Table 6.11
Analysis of Covariance: Mental Status

Source	DF	SS	MSS	F	P
Between Subjects	49	462.6400			
Covariate-AGE	1	56.5269		7.481	0.0088
P (Place)	1	50.9985	50.9985	6.750	0.0125
Subj w groups	47	355.1147	7.5556		
Within Subjects	100	123.3333			
T	2	4.8533	2.4267	2.181	0.1176
PT	2	11.6800	5.8400	5.249	0.0068
T x SwGps	96	106.8000	1.1125		

as high blood pressure (taking vital signs weekly or monitoring medication and diet), most RCFs do not provide mental health counseling for residents. Even the larger, more institutional facilities do not provide this component of care, except perhaps to refer residents for private counseling. Smaller homes are even less likely to recognize this problem or to assist a resident in finding needed mental health services. In addition, 20 percent of the respondents had been given a diagnosis of dementia. Since this sample was restricted to those capable of self-report, the actual incidence of mental function impairment among the RCF population may indeed be much higher.

QUANTITATIVE ANALYSIS

To test the six research hypotheses, an analysis of covariance was completed to examine the differences between the two samples on the research variables, controlling for the effects of age. The results of the analyses of covariance (ANCOVA) follow.

Hypothesis 1

From the data presented in Table 6.11, it appears that the main effect for place is significant. One could interpret that the RCF sample shows a significantly greater level of impairment in mental status as measured by the Short Portable Mental Status Questionnaire than does the community sample. When viewed with the data on the number of residents with a diagnosis of dementia, this finding is of special interest. Some confounding of the main effect, however, occurs as a result of a significant interaction effect of place and time. In Figure 6.2 it can be seen that, while the group scores differ, the groups themselves were changing over time (this variability is especially true of the RCF sample). (Except for the variable of social support, a higher score on the variable, or y axis, in Figures 6.2 through 6.6 indicates greater impairment or need for more assistance.) Thus the difference between groups may be due, in part, to the

Figure 6.2
Main Effects with Interactions: Mental Status

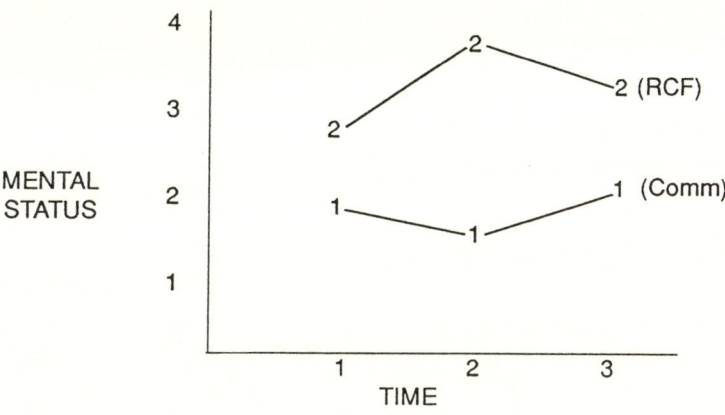

Table 6.12
Analysis of Covariance: Instrumental Activities of Daily Living

Source	DF	SS	MSS	F	P
Between Subjects	49	734.8267			
Covariate - AGE	1	305.4176	305.4176	38.764	0.0000
P (Place)	1	59.1044	59.1044	7.502	0.0087
Subj w groups	47	370.3046	7.8788		
Within Subjects	100	200.6668			
T	2	19.8933	9.9467	5.463	0.0056
PT	2	5.9733	2.9867	1.640	0.1979
T x SwGps	96	174.8000	1.8208		

changes within the groups over time. This change could be predicted from the earlier evidence of the changing nature of the RCF sample. It is of interest, however, that the RCF sample showed a slight increase in mental impairment score at time two. This rise could be seen as a response to the stress of adaptation to the new RCF environment during the first three months of the residents' stay. At six months, their scores approximated the original levels.

Hypothesis 2

The results of the ANCOVA shown in Table 6.12 present evidence that the RCF residents do show greater levels of impairment in the instrumental activities of daily living than the community sample. Again, however, some confounding of the main effects of place occur as the interaction effects with time approach

Figure 6.3
Main Effects with Interactions: Instrumental Activities of Daily Living

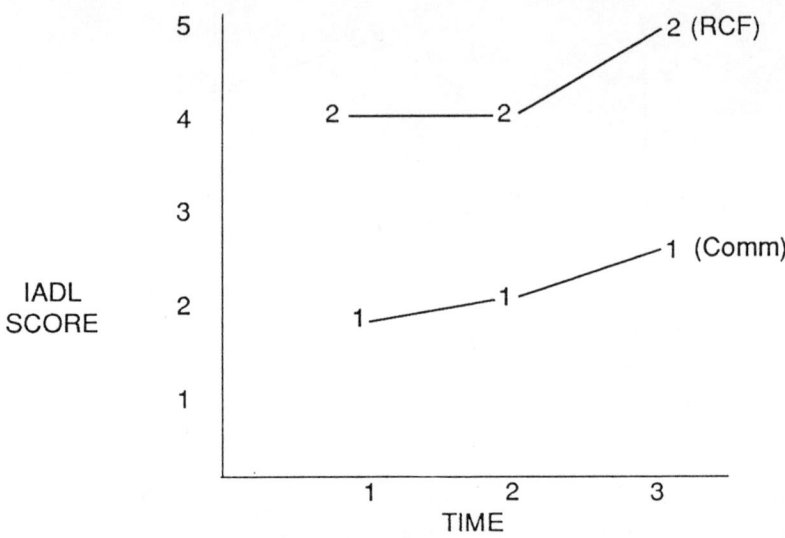

a significance level of 0.05. As in the discussion of mental status, it appears from Figure 6.3 that the within-groups change (especially in the RCF sample) contributes to the significance reported between groups. In particular, the RCF sample's scores have increased by the time of the third interview, indicating the need for more assistance with tasks such as using the telephone, shopping, meal preparation, housework, medications, and money management. It might be hypothesized that respondents report needing more assistance in these areas because it is provided by the RCF. Without available assistance, some of the residents might be able to perform these tasks. This hypothesis refers to the theories (Gray, 1976, 1977) that sheltered housing and care options may foster dependency in advance of actual need. Given the evidence of the frail and changing nature of the RCF sample, however, it may be that ability to perform these tasks has indeed declined because of changes in physical or mental status.

Hypothesis 3

From the F reported for the main effects of place in Table 6.13, it appears that the RCF residents were somewhat more impaired in the physical activities of daily living than their counterparts living in other community settings; the p value is, however, not significant at the .05 level. In addition, the main effects are confounded by the significant interaction effects reported for the factor of time (T) and place with time (PT). While these interaction effects make it difficult to interpret the main effects, Figure 6.4 provides some illumination. As with

Table 6.13
Analysis of Covariance: Physical Activities of Daily Living

Source	DF	SS	MSS	F	P
Between Subjects	49	372.0266			
Covariate - AGE	1	51.8189	51.8189	8.045	0.0067
P (Place)	1	17.4812	17.4812	2.714	0.1062
Subj w groups	47	302.7265	6.4410		
Within Subjects	100	58.6667			
T	2	4.4133	2.2067	4.183	0.0180
PT	2	3.6133	1.8067	3.425	0.0363
T x SwGps	96	50.6400	0.5275		

Figure 6.4
Main Effects with Interactions: Physical Activities of Daily Living (PADL)

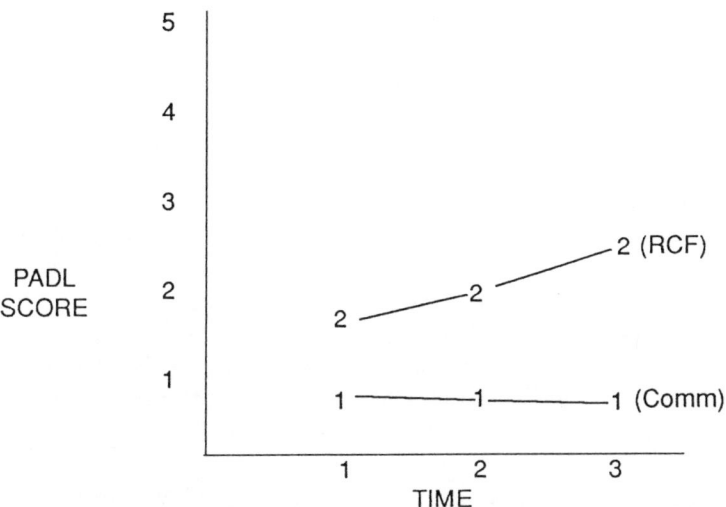

Note: The higher the PADL score, the less independent the resident.

the IADL scores, the RCF residents declined in their ability to perform the physical activities of daily living (PADL), such as bathing, dressing, grooming, maintenance of appearance, walking, and continence. It thus appears that the changes within the RCF sample over time contribute in some measure to the overall difference between groups. The descriptive analysis showed evidence that incidence of incontinence increased among the RCF sample. That increase and the fact that bathing and dressing assistance were provided by the facility may have contributed to the change in scores for this sample while the community sample remained virtually stable. The interaction effect of PT is not so readily interpreted and may be due in part to sampling error. With a larger sample and

Table 6.14
Analysis of Covariance: Affect Functioning

Source	DF	SS	MSS	F	P
Between Subjects	49	912.0067			
Covariate - AGE	1	15.7698	15.7698	0.829	0.3671
P (Place)	1	2.3420	2.3420	0.123	0.7272
Subj w groups	47	893.8950	19.0190		
Within Subjects	100	230.6667			
T	2	0.0933	0.0467	0.020	0.9802
PT	2	8.0400	4.0200	1.734	0.1807
T x SwGps	96	222.5333	2.3181		

less variance between the groups, a significant difference might be found in the physical activities of daily living.

Hypothesis 4

Table 6.14 presents the results of the ANCOVA for the variable Mental Health/Affect. The results show no significant main effects or interaction effects. Therefore one can assume no significant difference between the RCF sample and the community sample. While the descriptive analysis of RCF residents cited the high incidence of depression, no similar diagnostic data were available for the community sample. Therefore, while the descriptive data alone might indicate a greater level of depression in the RCF sample, the ANCOVA results do not confirm this hypothesis. In addition, the scale itself (SPES) is not merely a measure of depression but focuses on identifying functional psychiatric disorders of several types. It may be that a scale designed specifically to measure depression would be more appropriate in examining these populations.

Hypothesis 5

Table 6.15 presents the results of the ANCOVA for the variable Subjective Well-Being/Physical Health. No significant main effects or interaction effects appear. Therefore, the RCF residents seem not to rate their overall physical health significantly lower than do their counterparts in other housing settings.

Table 6.16 presents the results of the ANCOVA for the variable Subjective Well-Being/Mental Health. While significant values are reported for the main effect of place, some caution in accepting this result as confirmation of the hypothesis is in order. While the RCF sample shows higher scores on the scale measuring subjective mental health (Figure 6.5), the interaction effect of place and time within groups approaches significance and may indicate a significant error factor. It might be expected that the RCF residents, exhibiting greater mental impairment and having a large number with a primary diagnosis of

Table 6.15
Analysis of Covariance: Subjective Physical Health

Source	DF	SS	MSS	F	P
Between Subjects	49	276.7266			
Covariate - AGE	1	0.8854	0.8854	0.156	0.6944
P (Place)	1	9.6009	9.6009	1.695	0.1993
Subj w groups	47	266.2403	5.6647		
Within Subjects	100	110.6667			
T	2	1.6933	0.8467	0.760	0.4745
PT	2	1.9600	0.9800	0.879	0.4227
T x SwGps	96	107.0133	1.1147		

Table 6.16
Analysis of Covariance: Subjective Mental Health

Source	DF	SS	MSS	F	P
Between Subjects	49	224.1600			
Covariate - AGE	1	13.1183	13.1183	3.241	0.0782
P (Place)	1	20.8034	20.8034	5.140	0.0280
PT	47	190.2383	4.0476		
Within Subjects	100	145.3333			
T	2	4.6533	2.3267	1.676	0.1912
PT	2	7.3733	3.6867	2.655	0.0749
T x SwGps	96	133.3067	1.3886		

Figure 6.5
Main Effects with Interactions: Subjective Mental Health

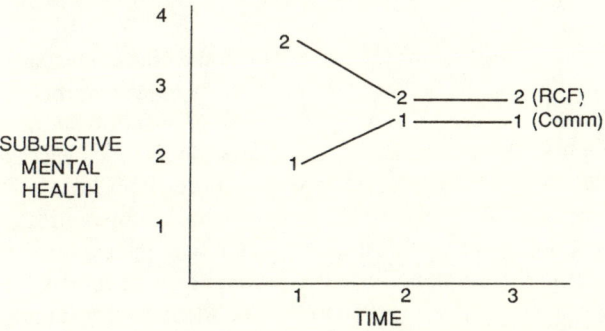

Table 6.17
Analysis of Covariance: Social Support

Source	DF	SS	MSS	F	P
Between Subjects	49	936.8333			
Covariate - AGE	1	1.8476	1.8476	0.093	0.7619
P (Place)	1	0.0594	0.0594	0.003	0.9566
Subj w groups	47	934.9263	19.8920		
Within Subjects	100	146.6668			
T	2	13.4400	6.7200	5.289	0.0066
PT	2	11.2533	5.6267	4.429	0.0144
T x SwGps	96	121.9733	1.2706		

depression, would rate their mental health lower than their counterparts in other settings. The awareness of failing mental capacity, which often prompts the move to a sheltered care facility, can be a source of fear and depression among older adults. These feelings might thus be reflected in a negative rating of overall mental health. The findings reported here seem to confirm this assessment but must be viewed with caution because of the interaction effects.

Hypothesis 6

Table 6.17 presents the results of the ANCOVA for the variable Social Support. No significant findings are reported for the main effect of Place, thus indicating no measurable difference between the two groups in the availability and effectiveness of their social support system. The interaction effects for the factors of Time and of Place with Time (PT) are statistically significant, however. Figure 6.6 shows that these within-group changes across time occur in both the RCF and the community sample.

DISCUSSION

While the results presented here should be viewed with some caution because of the small sample size and the statistical interaction effects, the data nevertheless do indicate that the residents of residential care facilities are more frail than their counterparts in alternative housing environments. Not surprisingly, the descriptive analysis suggests that the RCF population is older, more likely to move from another sheltered care setting to the RCF, more mentally impaired and takes more medications and needs more assistance with them than the population of older adults who remain in the community in private homes, apartments, or retirement settings. The forms of assistance given to RCF residents in this sample vary widely, but most receive assistance in multiple areas.

The results of the quantitative analysis suggest that the RCF respondents exhibit

Figure 6.6
Interaction Effects: Social Support

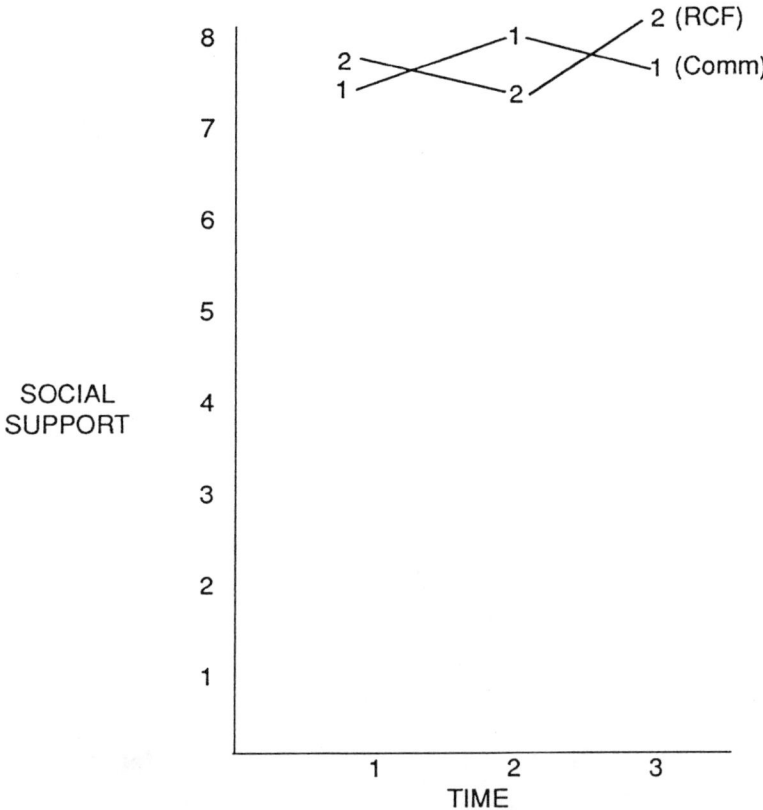

greater levels of mental impairment (as measured by the SPMSQ), need greater assistance with instrumental and physical activities of daily living, and rate their mental health lower than those older persons in the community sample. Of special interest is the fluctuating status of the RCF sample when compared to the community sample. For mental status, the RCF residents appeared to increase their levels of impairment at time 2, but they returned to previous levels by time 3. In the areas of physical and instrumental activities of daily living, the RCF sample show increased levels of impairment at each interview period, while subjective mental health scores for the RCF sample improved at time 2 and remained stable at time 3.

These findings have considerable policy implications for regulating and monitoring RCFs and for planning for those who expect to use these facilities in the future.

NOTE

1. To obtain information on the GATES or to review the instrument contact: Richard E. Cairl, Ph.D., Research Coordinator, Suncoast Gerontology Center, University of South Florida, Box 50, Tampa, FL 33612.

CHAPTER 7

Relationship Between Regulations/Industry and Needs of Consumers

It is obvious from the brief literature review of RCF users that current RCF residents would most closely resemble the nursing home population of previous decades. As the demand analysis in Chapter 2 underscored, more frail older persons than previously now reside in residential care alternatives, while nursing homes increasingly serve only the most severely impaired segment of the older population.

The demographic analysis in Chapter 6 verifies this earlier work. Compared to community residents, the residents of the RCF studied were older and more impaired and more likely to be female and widowed. In addition, some new information was provided regarding the prior residences of RCF consumers. Interestingly, fewer than expected came directly from their own homes or private apartments in the community. Almost half of the sample came from other assisted environments, such as retirement homes, foster care homes, or nursing homes. In addition, almost half had lived in the area for less than one year, implying that many residents might have moved to the vicinity to be closer to adult children.

The variables discriminating the RCF consumer from the community sample are primarily: (1) number of medications and inability to take them without assistance; (2) continence, with RCF residents having increasing difficulty with continence over time; (3) mental status, with almost one-fifth of the RCF residents having a diagnosis of dementia and showing significantly more impairment in mental status; and (4) increasing need over time for assistance with the instrumental activities of daily living.

While the sample for this study was small, and conclusions should be interpreted with caution, the findings still suggest some significant problems with current policies.

GENERALITY OF RCF REGULATIONS

First, RCFs in the state of Oregon are covered by regulations that leave a lot of "gray areas," as corroborated by state regulatory staff. Although RCFs legally cannot provide skilled nursing care, a broad range of possible care options exist between those for mobile persons and those for persons who need skilled nursing care. The specific question to be asked is whether RCFs can provide everything to all those who fall between these two extremes. I would argue that current requirements for staff ratios are inadequate to provide the range of care needed by frail older persons currently residing in RCFs. The types of assistance provided to RCF consumers (Chapter 6, Table 6.9) show that staff is needed in many ways. From the simplest task of reminding residents of meals and activities to multiple task assistance with showering, dressing, grooming, and continence, the level of care provided may vary from minimal for some residents to almost continual for others.

Second, current regulations do not reflect the changing intensity of service needs as the residents age during tenancy. This problem was especially noteworthy in this analysis as residents began to show increasing difficulty with continence, instrumental activities of daily living, and mental function. Continence, in particular, is a criterion that RCFs have often used to discriminate between those who are suitable for residence and those who need more assistance than they can provide. This study notes that continence became a problem for many residents over time. Will RCFs increasingly provide continence care or ask residents to move on to another level of care? If, as shown in this study, continence problems begin to arise within the first six months of residence, significant questions should be raised regarding long-term tenancy of residents and the impact of multiple relocations.

One solution proposed by owners and state staff alike is that a mix of residents should be maintained so that only a small percentage of the resident population at any one time will need intensive intervention to remain in the facility. This proposal, while ostensibly rational and feasible, poses several problems. The integration of more active, mentally alert residents with more physically frail and mentally impaired persons has been problematic. While some advocates have promoted the integration of elders with different abilities (Hiatt, 1982), others have noted the difficulty with such schemes (Cross, et al., 1979). Problems include resident dissatisfaction, inadequate design features to allow for greater impairment, inadequate staff to address increasing impairment, and the likelihood of a growing focus on those needing the most care, thus changing the nature of the facility.

While most previous research has focused on the aged who begin to show impairment in retirement facilities designed for the younger, more active older adult, the same factors may apply to the RCF setting. In addition, deterioration does not occur so predictably that a balance of impaired and less impaired can always be maintained. There is also the risk that as residents become more frail, more active older persons will be deterred from moving into such an environment.

If, however, this ideal integration were to occur, current regulations and design features would have to address this mix. In particular, the design of facilities critically affects the provision of adequate care and supervision, given current state requirements for staff and services. In the large new RCFs, which may house 100 to 150 individuals, several critical problems are evident as staff attempt to cope with a population who may show rapid decline in impairment or constantly fluctuating impairment.

For example, residents with increasing dysfunction in mental status may have difficulty in negotiating a large structure that has several floors, many halls, and numerous doorways that all look alike. Some new facilities focus on a unique design that allows the residents to have their own apartment. For those persons increasingly unable to find their way, the concept of their own space becomes difficult without clear visual cues, such as large signs or symbols with which to identify their corridor or apartment. Many facilities are unwilling to provide these highly visible cues, however, because they are seen as more like a nursing home (or do not fit in with the modern design envisioned for aesthetic and marketing purposes—a design to attract adult children searching for housing for an older parent). Whether these facilities can provide truly adaptable environments for older people with a range of physical and mental impairments remains to be seen.

Smaller facilities, particularly those run by one care provider in a private, single-family home adapted for care, may face other critical problems as residents age and show greater impairment. For example, the care provider who may cope well with one or two healthier, more alert residents and one very frail, mentally impaired, or incontinent resident may face stress and burn out when all three residents become significantly more impaired; such residents would need constant supervision to cope with wandering and other behavior associated with dementia, require assistance with all activities of daily living, and become increasingly immobile. While this scenario cites two extremes, state regulatory staffs' comments and the author's own experience in case management can validate the occurrence of such cases. Some of the smaller homes may also advertise their ability to provide for all levels of care when, in fact, the inadequate number and training of staff do not allow for the intensity of care needed by some residents. This problem is particularly true in homes where residents have come from hospitals, and still needing intensive assistance, are often discharged because of early discharge requirements under the DRG system. This problem is also especially difficult in facilities that care for patients with a diagnosis of Alzheimer's disease or other dementia.

MENTAL STATUS AS CRITICAL FACTOR

In particular, the level of mental impairment shown in the study sample and in the literature review and the problems with increasing mental dysfunction merit further discussion. While current staff ratios and policies for care make it difficult for facilities of all sizes to provide adequate physical care to a large number of frail older persons, the regulations are even less able to insure adequate supervision for the mentally impaired. In the current study, where only those residents capable of self-response were interviewed, almost one-fifth exhibited significant impairment in mental status. This finding indicates that a large percentage of the total RCF population probably shows some difficulty with daily function because of mental status; within that group some will exhibit extreme dysfunction requiring constant supervision and care. Current training requirements for administrators and direct care staff do not outline specific content areas. Overall, regulations focus on providing medical and personal care. Some direct regulatory intervention, in terms of training, design, and care for the mentally impaired, may be necessary to insure adequate levels of care for these residents.

Questions must also be asked about integrating the mentally alert with those exhibiting severe symptoms of dementia. With some forms of dementia, the impaired individual may exhibit aggressive and combative behavior, presenting a danger to staff and to other residents. One must certainly ask whether the RCF environment, designed with minimal staff requirements and promoted as an independent community alternative, is a suitable care option for persons exhibiting progressive behavioral problems associated with dementia.

In some instances, such as the increased documentation required for supervision of medications, the current regulations do address one aspect of the increasingly medical nature of RCFs; the increasingly stringent fire safety codes likewise reflect concern for the growing immobility of residents. These regulations do not, however, adequately address the levels of mental impairment among this population. For example, the Oregon fire marshal's requirements for RCFs currently do not allow for locked and secure outdoor areas from which residents cannot exit without staff assistance. While this sort of enclosed, secure area might be desirable to allow residents with dementia to walk without interference, it is viewed as an impediment to safety by one of the regulatory bodies. A locked and secure area most certainly reflects a more institutional character for the RCF and is one example of the move toward a more medical care alternative in the housing-care continuum. Again, the vagueness of this option poses unique dilemmas for regulatory intervention, as regulatory agencies strive to maintain the lower cost, alternative nature of such facilities in the face of increasingly frail populations demanding greater levels of care and supervision.

TRAINING

Training requirements for all staff also needs clarification in terms of the increasingly frail nature of the RCF population. As state staff have noted, when the regulations increase in number, and complexity and the care needs of residents simultaneously increase, the need for adequately trained staff becomes ever more critical to insure quality care. From the research reported here, administrative and direct care staff training should include care for the mentally impaired, continence care, and assessment of the changing care needs of a population exhibiting fluctuating mental and physical status. Current regulations do not adequately provide for the training of the administrator; staff training requirements are general in nature.

RESIDENT ASSESSMENT

The concept of resident assessment is important in any discussion of the appropriate placement of individuals in a level of housing or care. It is also important in monitoring the changing status of residents in RCFs. In the study reported here, a comprehensive functional assessment instrument (GATES), designed for use with older adults, was used to measure resident status over time. While the instrument yielded useful information on residents' mental status and ability to perform the physical and instrumental activities of daily living, it was not adequate to measure discernible differences in affect states, such as depression.

In addition, it did not address the residents' attitude toward the move to the RCF, a factor noted in other long-term care research as significant in determining the impact of relocation on subsequent resident status. The instrument also did not provide enough detailed information on the support system of residents. In particular, without the questions added by this researcher about previous location and length of residence in the community, it would have been difficult to determine the extent of the residents' community support system, which may augment the care provided by the facility.

The GATES instrument exhibits many of the inadequacies cited by Hiatt (1982) in her critique of existing assessment methodologies. As she noted:

Despite the number and variety of methods available for assessing the health and condition of older people, few of these adequately predict functioning. For example, we can measure eye sight or the presence of diseases, but this tells us all too little about the older person's ability to independently negotiate a particular type of home or to perform activities of daily living. One set of complications emerges because such evaluations are typically made in clinical settings and do not relate to experiences confronted in actual community programs or residences. Other difficulties arise because a person may appear independent or capable when judged. We simply do not have reliable, valid measures widely available and regularly administered to adequately reflect the capabilities of older people. (Pp. 38–39)

If it is difficult to measure capacity at any given point, it is even more difficult to adapt measures to provide an accurate picture of resident change over time. This need is particularly important in the RCF setting, where resident status is changing, often within a short period of time, and may require varying levels of care and supervision as a result.

In this study, the Mental Status Questionnaire, used in GATES to measure mental status, provides an excellent example of the problems with such methodologies. Although easy to administer, it is difficult to interpret well. While the overall score seems to reflect changes in mental status, it does not allow the user to identify how these impairments may prove problematic in the day-to-day environment. It is designed to measure aspects of both long- and short-term memory. In my study, it became obvious that, while a respondent might score in the very impaired range of the instrument (thus supposedly incapable of completing the remainder of the instrument), most respondents were clearly able to respond honestly and accurately to the remainder of the questionnaire items, particularly those related to their feelings.

In addition, the scale is generational and culture-specific. In other words, items that ask individuals to know the current date and day of the week may reflect the bias of working professionals. For those who have long been unemployed and may no longer participate in regularly planned social activities, not knowing the day and date may merely reflect a lack of necessity (or even depression), rather than declining mental function. In addition, the Short Psychiatric Evaluation Schedule used in GATES for measuring affect status may not accurately reflect the most common problem among the elderly, depression.

FUNDING: CRITICAL POLICY CONSTRAINT IN ADDRESSING MISMATCH

This review gives examples of a mismatch between the current regulations and facility designs and the needs of residential care consumers. To address this problem, certain changes are necessary on the part of both state regulatory agencies and the owners/administrators of facilities. Some of these changes have been noted, such as more stringent training requirements for staff and increased staff/resident ratios. Others, such as increased research and attention in the area of physical design, have been implied in the discussion of problematic design features for mentally impaired older adults. Some changes, such as a resolution of the locked, secure environment dilemma, indicate the need for recognizing the status of current RCF residents and changing regulations to accommodate these needs. Adequate resident assessment will require commitment by state staff to assess state-assisted clients; likewise, private proprietors must implement some form of assessment for private-pay residents.

All of these changes, however, require increased funding for implementation. Without administrative commitment to the residential care option, the likelihood of major funding increases is slight. Recent organizational changes undertaken to streamline the survey process may address some of the problems, but they will have limited effectiveness without adequate funding to implement the regulations for the changing nature of the RCF population. With neither appropriate sanctions for noncompliance nor federal reimbursement, private facilities have few incentives to assess clients to insure their ability to function and receive adequate care in the RCF setting.

The state has not been willing to address openly the medical and supervisory nature of RCFs, yet it tacitly acknowledges their growing involvement in providing injections, medication assistance, range-of-motion assistance, supervision, and continence care. The state has thus left open the possibility for facilities to say they can provide care to all. Without adequate funding to insure compliance with even the existing regulations, no mechanism exists to monitor the nature of care given in these facilities or to assess their appropriateness for a wide range of resident disabilities.

SUMMARY

The lack of clarity regarding the level of care provided in RCFs should be obvious by now. Current staff ratios (roughly one staff member on duty for each twenty residents) are clearly inadequate to provide the level of care indicated by the small study undertaken here. In addition, staff training requirements, building design, resident assessment, and funding levels do not reflect the growing frailty of RCF residents and the intensive medical and supervisory functions undertaken in these facilities.

Some may argue that further regulation will hamper the ability of these facilities to adapt to the range of impairments suffered by older persons or to provide a less costly and less restrictive environment for them. Unfortunately, the history of the nursing home industry has shown that, without intensive regulatory intervention (and even in spite of it), poor quality care is still commonplace. Why should we believe that a more humane and ethical value system underlies the RCF industry? A discussion of current and future trends may provide insight into possible avenues for growth and improvement in the residential care industry.

CHAPTER 8

Agenda for the Future: A Reformist View

This book initially discussed the role and function of residential care within the dichotomy of housing and health care, and noted its progression into the so-called "long-term care continuum." The place of the residential care option along this continuum has evolved largely as a function of the states' implementation of the Keys Amendment. At least in the state of Oregon, the degree of regulation and the commitment to reimbursement and support are functions of state policy.

In general, the growth of political capacity has been an important aspect of state government development in recent years. This change has significant implications for the way that states develop policies for the aging. It is particularly true for the residential care industry since few increases in the federal role for regulation and policy development are foreseen. As Lammers and Klingman (1984) have noted, "The gubernatorial, legislative, and administrative areas have all seen changes that enhance the capacity for states to design their own policies and to carry out policy implementation effectively" (p. 196). While increasing power may have been given to the state units, no source of increased funding has been forthcoming.

Other factors, including a climate of political openness, fiscal capacity, general policy liberalism, socioeconomic and demographic characteristics of the state's aging population, and levels of aging advocacy, may also affect the level and design of aging policy within a given state structure (Lammers & Klingman, 1984). As I have argued, an awareness of and commitment to residential care as an important alternative in the continuum of options for older persons is also a critical factor in the state's response. A review of current and proposed changes in the state of Oregon with references to other states may provide insight into the way of the future.

ACTUAL AND PROPOSED CHANGES IN OREGON'S RCF POLICIES AND REGULATIONS

One of the most critical changes affecting the licensing, regulating, and monitoring of residential care facilities in Oregon comes as part of a larger agency reorganization in long-term care. In July 1987 all long-term care administration and oversight, including the licensing and survey functions, were consolidated and placed under the Senior Services Division, Long Term Care Unit of the Department of Human Resources. These functions had previously been split between the Health Division and SSD. For example, the Health Division had been responsible for all federal certification (Title XVIII and Title XIX) of nursing homes; the Client Care Monitoring Units or CCMUs (which were moved to SSD in recent years) had been responsible for all Title XIX assessments and eligibility determination of clients.

Specifically, the four existing CCMUs and staff from the Health Division merged. They have assumed responsibility for certification, licensure, surveys, and client assessments for all nursing homes and for residential care facilities that are combined with nursing homes. The present registered nurse-surveyor within SSD is now assigned to the CCMU and will maintain responsibility for licensing, surveys, and client assessments for all other residential care facilities, with the exception of some rural facilities in the southern and easternmost parts of the state. In addition, this individual serves as the RCF specialist for all CCMUs, to be consulted in instances of unique or difficult problems. The merger also provides for a greater number of RCF residents to undergo periodic assessment by the review team. Where previously only Title XX recipients were assessed using state Form 360, a percentage of all residents will now be assessed, but the frequency of assessment may be as limited as every two years. Given the level of frailty and fluctuating status of residents noted in this research, these periodic assessments will not be adequate to assess the resident's functional status or appropriateness for a given facility. Infrequent assessment is particularly problematic given some state staff's assessment of Form 360, which they already judge inadequate for providing the type and amount of information needed to monitor increasingly frail residents. This judgment is especially significant since this same form will be used to determine clients' placement in the three classes of adult foster care.

The consolidation of all long-term care supervision appears to serve several functions, however. First, the state is thus decreasing the numbers of survey teams going into long-term care facilities. As one surveyor noted, "They'll be swamped one time by everybody rather than so many inspections over a given year or two." In addition, one state respondent indicated that the joint effort should decrease the "mixed messages" that administrators often get from different oversight agencies, which may note the same problem or deficiency in their review but give different advice on how to correct it or even set differing levels of improvement expected. Yet another bonus of the consolidation is what one surveyor described as "better utilization of the professional specialties." For example, the previous SSD survey team had only two members, a registered nurse and a program coordinator, who inspected when time allowed. The merger with the Health Division gives access to sanitarians, a dietician, and additional nursing staff.

This merger, however, clearly acknowledges the increasingly medical nature of residential care. Proposed changes in the regulations, while not specifically directed toward the medical aspects of care, reflect a concern with the level of care given and the qualifications of the caregivers. Thus, the legislature has mandated that "something be done about the rules and the rates."

Specifically, some proposals for change were considered during the 1987–88 legislative session. They include the following revisions in the rules for physical structure, services, programs, administration, and civil penalties.

1. *New Construction and Alterations*. Aimed primarily at facilities of sixteen beds or more, the rules, according to one committee member, "won't change what we have been requiring so much as it does spell them out clearly.... What the new rules will do is spell out in greater detail everything from the ventilation system to the kind of drinking fountain required." The new regulations address the size of resident rooms, increasing the total size per resident from 60 square feet to 100 square feet for single-bed rooms and 90 square feet per bed in multi-bed rooms. In addition, the regulations limit maximum capacity in multi-bed rooms to two residents. Toilet requirements, as proposed, are also increased, with one toilet serving no more than four beds and no more than two resident rooms: "Each resident shall have access to a toilet room without entering the general corridor area." Ironically, as one committee member remarked:

While we are providing more and more care, we have changed our whole concept of thinking from the time when everybody went down the hall someplace to go to the bathroom and that was acceptable, to the fact that we don't even want them to go out in the hallway to go to their bathing, and so on.... Our whole thinking about them has become a more private kind of arrangement... less institutional... more like an apartment arrangement... more like housing... and also many of the residents are now less mobile, less able to travel long distances to bath and toilet facilities.

The level of care dilemma continues, and, in recognition of the increasing frailty of residents, including the presence of more wheelchairs and walkers, proposed rules address corridor and door widths to allow for special devices.

2. *Services/Program/Administration*. State staff acknowledge that regulation changes need to address staffing requirements, both in numbers and in qualifications. In particular, educational requirements will likely be set for administrators, and the numbers of required direct care staff will increase slightly. Some clarification of the manner in which medications are handled will also be included. For example, one surveyor remarked that

we worked out many of the original regulations, both the program parts and the health sections with mental health when we were doing them. So, they have a real mental health flavor to them and some may not be appropriate for 70- and 80-year old people. . . . So we will refocus some of those things.

In addition, more specificity regarding admissions and discharges will be detailed.

3. *Civil Penalties.* The legislative council notified DHR that the civil penalties section of the administrative rules as written went beyond the legal mandate given to the agency. Therefore, a joint effort by DHR and the attorney general is underway to review and redesign this section. While Section 13 of the administrative rules for implementation of SB100 was vigorously opposed by providers, it is interesting to note that it has not been used for enforcement in a single instance since its passage. Several respondents noted, however, that it is more likely to be used in the coming years as residential care falls into the long-term care continuum outlined above in the section on the CCMU/Health Division merger. Health Division inspectors have been more inclined to use these penalties to insure compliance by nursing homes. As the two agencies merge for this function, the acceptance of Section 13's use as a sanction against repeated deficiencies in residential care facilities will probably grow.

What does the future hold for residential care in the state of Oregon? The administrative rules governing residential care continue to evolve and reflect the changing nature of residential alternatives. Proposals have also been discussed for moving reimbursement from a flat service rate to a client-based reimbursement system as is currently used in foster care. Under such a system, all residents would be evaluated; reimbursement would be based on level of care needed. This approach truly reflects a more medical approach to care, with client-based reimbursement growing out of the hospital and nursing home industries.

Other changes are afoot in the fire and safety realms. The National Fire Protection Association, for example, is attempting to establish fire safety guidelines based on individual resident ability to depart rather than on a system combining resident ability and characteristics of facility structure. State staff has expressed concern with this proposal by noting that it would require more constant monitoring of residents to assure their ability to depart a facility in case of an emergency. With residents who are frail and often exhibit fluctuations in physical and mental status, this consistent evaluation would be almost impossible.

Current practice requires a standard building structure based on general guidelines regarding the ability of residents to depart. As one surveyor noted, however, "At least the building is protected and if we maintain a certain standard for all facilities, then we don't have to be quite so fussy about whether the people in them are all fully ambulatory all the time." While none of those interviewed expected imminent change in fire safety to reflect this new approach, some acknowledged that the state fire marshal's office is interested in implementing such a system at the recommendation of the national association. Such a proposal is also likely to meet with support from many providers who feel that current regulations are a special impediment to the growth and/or maintenance of smaller facilities.

With the growing level of client impairment in residential care facilities, some attention will have to be given to increasing reimbursement rates for more demanding care. A demonstration project is currently underway to test the viability of placing state assistance clients in more expensive, private care facilities by adding additional reimbursement for "special services" over and above the required care. While recognizing the project as a unique approach to increasing reimbursement without seeking additional state appropriations, state program staff expressed reservations concerning the use of such a system. In effect, the facility, in looking for extra services to provide in order to house state assistance clients, could "cross that fine line" between residential care and intermediate nursing care.

By far, the most critical change occurring in the residential care industry in Oregon will result from new state regulations that set up yet another level of care. The term *assisted living* has been given to this level. According to one state staff person, these facility regulations will focus more on care than do current RCF requirements. The old RCF designation will remain. While the difference between the two is not yet clear, staff mentioned ideals such as "incorporating a philosophy of independence and choice." As expected, many current RCF providers interviewed felt that the new designation was not needed. Some expressed a long-held belief that the state just needs to provide better reimbursement for existing RCFs to bring them to a desired standard. Adding another layer in the care continuum only confuses (or masks) the issue. Others in the field believe that the new assisted living designation has come from private developers with a special interest in this form of housing. This change may reflect more concern with the frailty of residents described here and as such may be a positive change for insuring quality care. Developments in regulations should be evaluated in this light.

Most state staff members who were interviewed believed that no additional major interventions would come from the federal government in the area of residential care. Only one person suggested that the federal government might go beyond recommended areas of regulation coverage to mandate certain aspects of care. Specifically, it was suggested that the federal government might begin to mandate that facilities accept a certain percentage of Title XIX clients in a manner close to that now prescribed for nursing homes.

As more facilities turn to providing licensed residential care, including free-standing structures and those connected with retirement and nursing homes, adequate regulation and oversight become increasingly important. Whether the reorganization of the long-term care unit can accomplish this goal without significant increases in funding remains to be seen. As Estes (1979) pointed out, policy makers have often called for better coordination among limited services to avoid the more basic questions surrounding adequate funding. Merely making inadequate services more efficient will not address the fundamental lack of resource commitment.

Whether residential care can evolve to meet the growing frailty of its residents is also an unanswered question. One state surveyor, peering into the future, suggested that residential care is here to stay and predicted that

> we are going to see more retirement homes built, and more great big residential care facilities built.... I have always thought that the trend is going to be for the retirement homes to have an ICF, plus residential care ... and nursing homes will be only for skilled care. In residential care, I think the word "care" is going to stay in there and be the focus.

The impact of the demise of smaller, home-based residential facilities is also difficult to determine. Perhaps that role is being assumed by foster care homes, a possibility that in turn brings forth a wealth of questions and need for research.

One must ask whether the changes proposed for Oregon will have any measurable impact on addressing the problems in residential care. The reorganization described here is one in a long line of coordination strategies proposed for improving services to the elderly. Given previous federal, state, and local attempts to improve service by better coordination in lieu of better funding or more creative interventions, the prognosis for real improvement is poor. The continued focus on the physical plant and the medical aspects of care also overlooks the need for a sense of community and self-worth by residents—the more difficult to measure quality-of-life variables.

Form 360, currently in use to assess the appropriate placement of residents in RCFs, needs to be reviewed as an adequate measure for the changing functional status of frail residents. Although a great deal of development time and numerous revisions have been invested in this instrument, some objective review of its usefulness for this purpose should be undertaken. In particular, its ability to measure change over time should be examined.

In addition, without commitment from state administrative staff and from the larger public regarding the validity and desirability of residential care facilities, it is difficult to imagine real change occurring in the near future.

THE NATIONAL PICTURE

In reporting the major national study of residential care alternatives to date, Mor et al. (1986) emphasize that "the national scope and size of the residential care options is substantial, meriting considerably more research attention than has been accorded it to date" (p. 414). In addition, the national study and the present research raise critical questions regarding the best type of residential facility for the increasingly frail, dependent aged who heretofore have been admitted to nursing homes. Mor et al. (1986) examined the institutional and the family type of RCF, as well as RCFs regulated by departments of health or by integrated state programs (usually welfare, social service, or mental health). Significant differences were found between small and large facilities and among those regulated by various types of state agencies. Mor's findings reflect many of the issues uncovered in this book, including inadequate staff training; physical design considerations; difficulty in monitoring the many small, decentralized, and often less regulated family foster homes; and possible deleterious effects of using RCFs (and especially the smaller homes) as an outlet for the spillover effect of DRGs.

In addition, the more institutional, medical model most characteristic of the larger facilities may not be a relevant alternative to continued care at home for older persons who exhibit only moderate social and psychological impairments and have few social supports. These facilities may more appropriately meet the increased demand for nursing home beds. In particular, they may adapt their facilities to allow for intermediate care patients no longer provided for under federal nursing home reimbursement. Indeed, one can speculate that RCF care might become a reimburseable level of care under Medicaid in the future. Already some states, such as California, are considering allowing RCFs reimbursement under a state long-term care insurance program.

Other states are also implementing changes that affect the RCF industry. Minnesota, for example, incorporated board and care into their long-term care system by giving it the designation of Intermediate II (ICF II). In 1986, the state adopted a case-mix system of reimbursement based on assessments of residents' abilities in ADLs. Using a system similar to Oregon's, Minnesota uses a standardized assessment form to determine a client's level of care. California is also considering implementing a system of three levels of care for residential alternatives. This three-tiered regulatory and reimbursement structure for residential care facilities for the elderly (RCFE) would allow residents to remain at this level of care (versus nursing home care) as their needs increase. Similar experiments in other states seem likely.

A RETURN TO THEORY

Several issues of theoretical importance have been raised by this analysis. Now that some specifics of the residential care industry have been examined, a return to these issues is in order.

Models of Care

The concepts of the dichotomy and the continuum are both inadequate to describe the current situation of older persons in long-term care. The model that most closely reflects the range of housing and care options needed is the continuum. Yet even this model does not reflect accurately the realities of aging.

The continuum model has assumed movement along the range of options as an older person experiences increasing needs for assistance with daily living and with medical care. The literature reflects, and this study has shown, however, that, even in the RCF, individuals do not move along to the next level of care in a different setting. Rather, they become more dependent in their current living environment. More explicitly, the continuum exists even within each care option.

Given the research on the impact of relocation, which seems more severe as an individual reaches higher levels of impairment, the continuum model may be outmoded and even undesirable. It may reflect an ideal where each individual would move along to the most appropriate setting as increments of frailty accumulate. Yet the costs associated with moving, costs that are both physical and psychological, may realistically imply that each level in the continuum should be designed so that individuals may move to one setting offering some assistance and remain there, adding services as needed.

The financial costs associated with insuring the multiple levels of care required to meet the needs of the RCF population may be prohibitive, however. Even if regulation existed to provide more clearly for the frail nature of RCF residents, the impact on the industry as a whole could be inhibiting. This study, then, has perhaps served to delineate more clearly the bind described earlier—that of insuring adequate care without regulating the industry out of existence.

The Role of Regulation

This study has raised a range of issues regarding the regulatory process. It has highlighted the ineffectiveness of relying on regulatory precedent that does not fit present needs. In other words, it only bolsters Bardach and Kagan's (1982) statement that "there is no general theory of regulatory design with sufficient power to furnish good guidance on particular questions" (p. 302). Lacking "good guidance," bureaucrats at both the state and federal level have relied on the history of regulation in nursing home care, where claims of regulatory unreasonableness have been common.

So, what constitutes reasonable regulation in the growing residential care industry? I have argued that some increase in regulation is necessary to insure adequate care for the frail population residing in these facilities. Thus, if regulation is to persist, "and if reform cannot be brought about by simple, global solutions, the challenge for government is the far more complex one of selecting the appropriate regulatory implements more wisely and of developing the competence to regulate more reasonably and responsibly" (Bardach & Kagan, 1982, p. 301).

A general theory of regulatory reform, then, would leave open a variety of strategies from which to choose. Perhaps several strategies could complement one another. In the case of residential care, creative regulation would involve reliance on more than one mechanism. It might, for instance, draw on the unused but already mandated role of the ombudsman in reviewing quality of care and compliance in RCFs. A 1978 amendment to the Older Americans Act "recommended" that nursing home ombudsman programs include advocacy for residents of board and care/residential care facilities. The ombudsman program, even in the monitoring of nursing homes, has so far proven ineffectual. The potential for such a program, however, with its ability to provide public visibility for both good and bad facilities has been grossly underutilized.

With both the ombudsman program and the calls for improvement of the regulatory process, adequate resources are essential to hire and train more competent inspectors and advocates. Rather than add regulations, a first effort at reform might more reasonably call for adequate resources to implement existing regulations and for a wider range of options for the regulator and the ombudsman in their attempts to increase compliance. Given that demands for budget increases are met with calls for constraint, Bardach and Kagan (1982) noted that regulatory agencies "might rely more on educational strategies, mandatory disclosure regulations, or assistance to private litigants rather than invest all their resources in more expensive (and probably more unreasonable) direct regulation and enforcement" (p. 305).

Whatever the reform chosen, "the central tenet of an acceptable public philosophy of regulation must . . . be the affirmation that norms of social responsibility originate in society or in public opinion, and not in the state" (p. 319). The inescapable conclusion is that public sentiment must validate the importance of quality housing, social welfare, and medical care for older people in order for regulation to be effective. Only with the support of the community can real reform occur. Only with a commitment to the welfare of older adults will pressure be brought on policy makers to provide adequate resources with which to provide care and monitor its quality over time.

Any policy choice demands that the true character of these facilities be acknowledged. If, as Mor et al. (1986) implied, the residential care industry reflects within itself a continuum of care from moderately supervised housing to intermediate nursing care, the regulatory agencies monitoring these facilities will have to structure policies and regulations that reflect the range and intensity of care provided in them. These regulations will need to be structured to adequately insure that the quality of care is maintained.

Developing such standards will be a challenge in the current climate of cost containment and focus on deregulation. Predicting the evolution of protective regulation in the RCF industry is therefore difficult. As Bardach and Kagan (1982) pointed out, the United States has entered an era in which the costs of regulation are a matter of concern for liberals as well as conservatives. The nature of regulation may be changing in response. They hypothesized that "more and more regulatory agencies, recognizing the excesses of legalistic regulations, will institute strategies of flexible enforcement and will try to revise their rules and regulations as well" (p. 185). The regulatory agencies addressing the RCF industry should examine the history of their efforts in similar fields and acknowledge the costs associated with intensive intervention, such as those that occurred in the nursing home industry. They might as a result temper the stringency of the developing RCF regulations to reflect greater reasonableness in this long-term care option. Serious questions remain, however, about the hazards of being reasonable.

If residential care continues to grow as an option for both housing and long-term care of the dependent elderly, a clearer understanding of its nature and its residents is needed.

The Issue of Costs

This discussion has raised questions regarding the costs associated with insuring adequate enforcement of regulations in RCFs as well as the costs associated with providing care to a more frail population. A further critical question concerns the assumptions regarding the costs of residential care. If the custodial housing model is assumed, as it seems to have been in the past, then the costs of providing housing and care should presumably be less than those of nursing homes or health care per se. As this study has shown, however, those in residential care may need intensive intervention that may not be directly health-related. For example, residents who have Alzheimer's disease or some other severe form of dementia may still require an immense amount of supervision; the care may still require costly staff time to administer. The current levels of funding and staffing requirements seem not to recognize that intensive custodial care may be as costly and require as much staff as medical intervention. The type of staff needed may differ, but greater numbers of staff members may be needed. Recognition of this reality could produce a more realistic budgetary analysis at the state and federal level.

The costs associated with upgrading personnel in residential care facilities are also problematic. Interestingly, recent federal requests for proposals have targeted developing educational programs for adult foster care providers. Some of the problems previously encountered in educational efforts for this group might provide insight into approaches for RCF staff. Certainly a similar federal commitment to education for RCF providers in larger facilities is needed. Federal grants to states and to educational institutions are one mechanism by which further upgrading of personnel can occur.

NEED FOR ADDITIONAL RESEARCH

This study has posed many questions and, in providing answers to some, has clarified the need for further examination of the others. Specifically, further research is needed in the following areas:

1. Effective client assessment—the ability to document the current users of residential care, their characteristics, and needs—is the first step in addressing the true nature of the RCF and the type of residents it is best suited to serve. Without knowledge of the consumers, any policies for these facilities will develop in an environment where: (a) special interests can dominate; (b) blanket and

generalized policies make it difficult for small facilities to survive but do not adequately address the level of care provided in larger, more medical facilities; (c) quality of care and well-being of residents will be difficult to measure; and (d) the training needs of RCF staff may or may not be adequately addressed. Without accurate information regarding the medical care needs of RCF residents, one cannot begin to measure the ability of providers to give adequate care. Accurate assessment requires the refinement of existing instruments or the development of new instruments to measure physical and mental status of RCF residents. Specifically, since a large percentage may be incapable of accurate self-report, effective observational techniques will be needed to determine the residents' functional abilities.

The role of testing and screening of residents at all levels of care deserves greater attention. The proliferation of instruments for testing functional capacity has still not produced instruments that adequately measure an older person's ability to function in a given environment, nor have the policy implications of testing and/or retesting of residents been adequately explored. The policy issues include costs associated with multiple assessments, personnel needs to implement assessment in both public and private facilities, and the rights to privacy and personal control on the part of residents who will be measured. Moreover, if residents do not really move along a continuum, then the purpose of functional assessments must be reexamined. These instruments have been developed primarily to place individuals in a given level of care to keep them from an inappropriate one. If, however, the purpose changes to one of measuring an individual's ability to function over time in a given facility, the structure and validity of the instruments must be reanalyzed.

2. More attention must be focused on the impact of current reimbursement levels and regulations on the supply of residential homes, particularly those serving the low-income older person. If current regulations make it difficult for the smaller, less costly private home to maintain an economic incentive, then policy development must address this issue to insure care for all older persons regardless of income. One possible option is a federal and state loan program to insure the development and operation of facilities serving the low- and middle-income resident; another is two-level (or more) designations for residential care facilities to reflect the range of services currently provided. These designations could mirror the schemes in England that allow for sheltered housing and extra-sheltered housing to allow for the increasing needs of dependent elders.

3. Research must examine each state's style and level of intervention in the RCF industry to determine if common issues, problems, and solutions can be identified. This statement hardly represents a call for uniformity, but the size of the industry indicates some general trends from which we may learn more clearly the role of the RCF and methods for insuring quality care in these facilities. If this analysis were undertaken, RCF definitions and terminology could be made comparable across the states so that industry-wide research could be undertaken

with some greater degree of confidence. Concomitantly, federal efforts could focus on including these facilities, with uniform definitions, in national census and health surveys.

4. The impact of rapid turnover in RCF administrative and direct-care staff deserves attention. The causes and effects of this phenomenon should be examined and every effort should be made to insure that policies and regulations reflect a concern with the effect on RCF residents. The nursing home industry may provide clues about the causes of turnover and may offer some mechanisms for improvement.

5. Designers and environmental gerontologists should focus their attention on the appropriate size and design of residential facilities for the frail elderly. These efforts would ideally identify environmental factors critical to the care of the mentally impaired older adult and detail the pros and cons of various sizes and designs of small and large residential care facilities. This type of specificity would contribute to more appropriate placement of clients and even indicate staff training needs in various types of facilities. An additional design and policy issue is the question of the adaptability of residential care facilities. That is, should the facilities be designed to accommodate residents at the most impaired end of the functional scale? What are the cost implications of such design? What impact would such designs have on smaller facilities less able to meet these requirements? Again, knowing more clearly the characteristics of the RCF population would add to the policy makers' ability to determine what the design criteria should be and to assess the cost-effectiveness of requiring such modifications.

6. Research efforts should work to assess the impact of integrating the levels of frailty seen among the RCF population. Implications for the residents' satisfaction, health, and mental status, as well as the staff's ability to cope with a broad range of impairments, should be analyzed.

7. Finally, a critical dialogue should be undertaken about the ideology of community care. Questions must be raised about the emphasis placed on family-like care. The effects on consumers should be studied. For example, research that examines resident satisfaction with forms of care must go beyond exploring preferences. The effects on providers also deserve attention. For example, reliance on the ideology of familism has serious implications for women, who provide the bulk of care in both institutional and community settings. As Dalley (1988) has noted, community care may in fact take women from low-paying jobs in institutional settings and place them in home-occupations where they still receive low pay and also lose benefits, bargaining power, or union representation. In addition, reviewing the experiences of the deinstitutionalization movement and the consequences of community care for the mentally impaired may provide insights that can guide the growth of community care alternatives for the elderly.

FINAL NOTES

The residential care facility, in all its existing forms, creates seemingly contradictory needs and demands, similar to those seen in other congregate residences for older persons. That is, residents of these facilities reflect the progressive need for medical and support services in conflict with the ability and desire to maintain an active, independent life. The primary question remains whether one facility can fulfill these contradictory aims.

As this study has shown, residential care facilities increasingly provide care for a more impaired, dependent population, for whom independence and activity may be severely limited. Current policy, however, reflects a desire to maintain some aspects of more independent living in these facilities. As noted in a recent study, "a better understanding of the boundaries between medical and non-medical needs of the long-term care population would help to clarify who can most effectively be cared for in the various community-based and facility-based programs" (California Health and Welfare Agency, 1988). Resolution of these issues is a major challenge for policy makers and aging advocates concerned with long-term care in the coming decades. The goal should be not only to provide a range of options within the continuum of care, but to insure that quality care is provided in each type of housing and care arrangement. Maintaining a balance between imposing regulation and fostering expansion of a needed long-term care option is clearly the challenge set for federal and state policy makers.

In sum, it is my hope that the research reported here will inspire and stimulate activity in addressing some of the critical issues raised and thus lead to policies to insure quality housing and care options for older people who live in the space we call long-term care.

References

Abrams, M. (1978). Beyond three-score and ten: A first report. *Age concern* (Manchester, England: National Corporation for the Care of Old People and Age Concern. [England]).

Allison, G. T. (1971). *Essence of decision: Explaining the Cuban missile crisis*. Boston, MA: Little, Brown.

Anderson (Eustis), N. N. Patten, S. K., & Greenberg, J. N. (1980). *A comparison of home care and nursing home care for older persons in Minnesota*. Minneapolis, MN: University of Minnesota, Hubert H. Humphrey Institute of Public Affairs and the Center for Health Services Research.

Baggett, S. (1983). Historical perspective of the long term care facility. In M. O. Hogstel (Ed.), *Management of personnel in long term care* (pp. 52–77). Bowie, MD: Robert J. Brady.

Bardach, E., & Kagan, R. A. (1982). *Going by the book: The problem of regulatory unreasonableness*. Philadelphia: Temple University.

Barney, J. L. (1973). *Patients in Michigan's nursing homes: Who are they? How are they? Why are they there?* Ann Arbor: University of Michigan-Wayne State University (Institute of Gerontology).

Bovbjerg, R. R., & Holahan, J. (1982). *Medicaid in the Reagan era: Federal policy and state choices*. Washington, DC: the Urban Institute.

Bradshaw, B., Vonderhaar, W., Keeney, V., Tyler, L., & Harris, S. (1976). Community based residential care for the minimally impaired elderly: A survey analysis. *Journal of the American Geriatrics Society, 24*(9), 423–429.

Brody, E. (1969). Follow-up study of applicants and non-applicants to a voluntary home. *Gerontologist, 9*(3), 187–196.

Brody, E., Johnsen, P., Fulcomer, M., & Lang, A. (1983). Women's changing roles and help to elderly parents: Attitudes of three generations of women. *Journal of Gerontology, 38*(5), 597–607.

Brody, E., & Schoonover, C. (1986). Patterns of parent-care when adult daughters work and when they do not. *Gerontologist, 26*(4), 372–381.

Brody, S. J., & Persily, N. A. (1984). *Hospitals and the aged: The new old market.* Rockville, MD: Aspen Systems.
Brown, L. D. (1983a). Health policy in the Reagan administration: A critical appraisal. *Bulletin of the New York Academy of Medicine, 59*(1), 31–49.
Brown, L. D. (1983b). *New policies, new politics.* Washington, DC: The Brookings Institution.
Butler, A., Oldman, C., & Greve, J. (1983). *Sheltered housing for the elderly: Policy, practice, and the consumer.* Boston, MA: George Allen & Unwin.
Butler, L. H., & Newacheck, P. W. (1981). Health and social factors relevant to long term care policy. In J. Meltzer, F. Farrow, & H. Richman (Eds.), *Policy options in long-term care.* Chicago: University of Chicago.
Byerts, T. O., & Heller, T. (1985). *Longitudinal research on congregate public housing: Executive summary.* Chicago, IL: University of Illinois at Chicago, College of Architecture.
Bytheway, B., & James, L. (1978). *The allocation of sheltered housing: A study of theory, practice, and liaison.* Swansea, Wales: University College of Swansea.
Cairl, R. E., Pfeiffer, E., & Keller, D. (undated). *Geriatric assessment testing and evaluation system comprehensive assessment form.* Tampa, FL: Suncoast Gerontology Center, University of Florida.
California Health and Welfare Agency. (1988). *A study of California's publicly-funded long-term care program.* Sacramento, CA: Author.
Cantor, M. H. (1979). Neighbors and friends: An overlooked resource in the informal support system. *Research on Aging, 1,* 434–463.
Center for the Study of Social Policy (1988). *Completing the long term care continuum: An income supplement strategy.* Washington, DC: Author.
Certificate and order for filing administrative rules with the secretary of State (U.S.), 410–04–002, August 14, 1978.
Chelimsky, E. (1985). *GAO study to identify issues pertaining to the impact of prospective payment system on long-term care.* From letter to the Honorable John Heinz. U.S. General Accounting Office, Feb. 1985.
Chubb, J. E. (1985). Federalism and the bias for centralization. In J. E. Chubb & P. E. Peterson (Eds.), *The new direction in American politics* (pp. 273–306). Washington, DC: The Brookings Institution.
Coe, M., Wilkinson, A., & Patterson, P. (1986). *Preliminary evidence on the impact of DRG's: Dependency at discharge study* (Final Report, HCFA Grant #18-C-98862/0-01). Beaverton, OR: Northwest Oregon Health Systems.
Cross, D., Mattson, L., Gray, K., Pyrek, J., & Carrol, K. (1979, November). *The impact of integrated groups of alert and confused elderly.* Paper presented at the 32nd annual meeting of the Gerontological Society, Washington, DC.
Dalley, G. (1988). *Ideologies of caring: Rethinking community and collectivism.* London: Macmillan Education.
Davis, K. (1984). Medicare reconsidered. In D. Yaggy (Ed.), *Health care for the poor and elderly: Meeting the challenge* (pp. 77–96). Durham, NC: Duke University.
Davis, S. M. & Gibbin, M. J. (1971). An areawide examination of nursing home use, misuse, and nonuse. *American Journal of Public Health, 61*(6), 1146–1155.
Dick, H., Friedsam, H., & Martin, C. (1964). Residential patterns of aged persons prior to institutionalization. *Journal of Marriage & Family, 26*(1), 96–98.
Dittmar, N. D., & Smith, G. P. (1983). *Evaluation of board and care homes: Summary of survey procedures and findings.* Denver, CO: Denver Research Institute.

Dunlop, B. D. (1976). *Determinants of long-term care facility utilization by the elderly: An empirical analysis.* (Working Paper.) Washington, DC: The Urban Institute.
Dunlop, B. D. (1979). *The growth of nursing home care.* Lexington, MA: Lexington.
Eckert, J. K., Namazi, K. H., & Kahana, E. (1987). Unlicensed board and care homes: An extra-familial living arrangement for the elderly. *Journal of Cross-Cultural Gerontology, 2*, 377–393.
Estes, C. L. (1979). *The aging enterprise.* San Francisco, CA: Jossey-Bass.
Estes, C. L. (1982). Austerity and aging. *International Journal of Health Services, 12*(4), 573–584.
Estes, C. L., & Gerard, L. (1983). Governmental responsibility: Issues of reform and federalism. In C. L. Estes, R. J. Newcomer, & Associates, *Fiscal austerity and aging* (pp. 41–58). Beverly Hills, CA: Sage.
Estes, C. L., & Lee, P. R. (1985). Social, political, and economic background of long term care policy. In C. Harrington, R. J. Newcomer, C. L. Estes, & Associates, *Long term care of the elderly: Public policy issues* (pp. 17–39). Beverly Hills, CA: Sage.
Estes, C. L., Newcomer, R. J., & Associates. (1983). *Fiscal austerity and aging.* Beverly Hills, CA: Sage.
Eustis, N., Greenberg, J., & Patten, S. (1984). *Long-term care for older persons: A policy perspective.* Monterey, CA: Brooks/Cole.
Feder, J. (1983). Effects of changing federal health policies on the general public, the aged, and disabled. *Bulletin of the New York Academy of Medicine, 59*(1), 41–49.
Feller, B. A. (1983). Americans needing help to function at home. In *National Center for Health Statistics: Advanced Data, 92* (DHHS Pub. No. PHS 83–1250). Hyattsville, MD: U.S. National Center for Health Statistics.
Fischer, D. H. (1978). *Growing old in America.* New York: Oxford University.
Fisher, C. R. (1980). Differences by age groups in health care spending. *Health Care Financing Review, 1*(4), 65–90.
Freeland, M. S., & Schendler, C. E. (1983). National health expenditure growth in the 1980's: An aging population, new technologies, and increasing competition. *Health Care Financing Review, 4*(3), 1–59.
George Washington University. (1969). *The evolution of long term care in the United States: A study of nursing homes and related facilities.* Monograph No. 1. Washington, DC: Author.
Gioglio, G., & Jacobsen, R. (1984). *Demographic and service characteristics of the rooming home, boarding home, and residential health care facility population in New Jersey.* Trenton, NJ: Bureau of Research, Evaluation and Quality Assurance, Division of Youth and Family Services, Department of Human Services.
Glenn, K. (1985). Hospital continuing care arrangements. *Washington Report on Medicine and Health, 39*(19), 4.
Goffman, E. (1961). *Asylums.* Garden City, NY: Doubleday.
Gollay, E., Freedman, R., Wyngaarden, M., & Kurtz, N. R. (1978). *Coming back: The community experiences of deinstitutionalized mentally retarded people.* Cambridge, MA: Abt Associates, Inc.
Gray, J.A.M. (1976). Housing: Is the emphasis on sheltered housing right? *Modern Geriatrics, 7*(2), 9–11.

Gray, J.A.M. (1977). Housing for elderly people: Heaven, haven and ghetto. *Housing Monthly, 12*(6), 12–13.

Greenberg, J. N., & Ginn, A. (1979). A multivariate analysis of the predictors of long term care placements. *Home Health Services Quarterly, 1*(1), 75–99.

Gubrium, J. F. (Ed.). (1973). *The myth of the golden years.* Springfield, IL: Thomas.

Gubrium, J. F. (1975). *Living and dying at Murray Manor.* New York: St. Martin's.

Gutkin, C. (1980). *Domiciliary care for adults in Pennsylvania.* Doctoral Thesis, Florence Heller School for Graduate Studies in Social Welfare. Boston, MA: Brandeis University.

Gutkin, C., & Sherwood, S. (1979). *First Pennsylvania domiciliary care home report: An evaluation of the Pennsylvania Domiciliary Care Program* (Mimeo Report. DHEW Contract #130–76–12). Boston, MA: Hebrew Rehabilitation Center for the Aged.

Harlow, K. W., & Wilson, L. B. (1985). *DRG's and the community-based long term care system.* Paper presented to Committee on Education and Labor Subcommittee on Human Resources, U.S. House of Representatives. Dallas, TX: University of Texas Health Science Center at Dallas, Southwest Long Term Care Gerontology Center.

Harmon, C. (1982). *Board and care: An old problem, new resource of long-term care.* Washington, DC: Center for the Study of Social Policy.

Harrington, C., Estes, C. L., Lee, P. R., & Newcomer, R. J. (1985). State policies on long term care. In C. Harrington, R. J. Newcomer, C. L. Estes, & Associates, *Long term care of the elderly: Public policy issues* (pp. 67–88). Beverly Hills, CA: Sage.

Harrington, C., & Swan, J. H. (1985). Institutional long term care services. In C. Harrington, R. Newcomer, C. L. Estes, & Associates, *Long term care of the elderly: Public policy issues* (pp. 153–176). Beverly Hills, CA: Sage.

Harrington, C., Newcomer, R. J., Estes, C. L., & Associates. (1985). *Long term care of the elderly: Public policy issues.* Beverly Hills, CA: Sage.

Hendricks, J., & Hendricks, C. D. (1977). *Aging in mass society: Myths and realities.* Cambridge, MA: Winthrop.

Henry, J. (1963). *Culture against man.* New York: Random House.

Hiatt, L. (1982). Grouping elders of different abilities. In R. D. Chellis, J. F. Seagle, B. M. Seagle (Eds.), *Congregate housing for older people* (pp. 27–49). Lexington, MA: Lexington.

Hillhaven Foundation. (1980). *Final report of the National Conference on long term care issues.* Washington, DC: Hillhaven Foundation.

Holahan, J. F. (1983). The medically needy and needy. *Bulletin of the New York Academy of Medicine, 59*(1), 59–68.

Holahan, J. F., & Stassen, M. (1980). *Long term care demonstration projects: A review of recent evaluations* (Working Papers 1227–2). Washington, DC: The Urban Institute.

Holmes, D., Teresi, J., & Holmes, M. (1983). Differences among black, Hispanic, and white people in knowledge about long-term care services. *Health Care Financing Review, 5*(2), 51–67.

Israel, L., Kozarevic, D., & Sartorius, N. (with collaboration of the World Health Organization). (1984). *Source book of geriatric assessment, Vol. 1: Evaluations in gerontology.* New York: Karger.

Janicki, M. P., Mayeda, T., and Epple, W. A. (1982). *A report on the availability of group homes for persons with mental retardation in the United States.* Albany, NY: New York State Office of Mental Retardation and Developmental Disabilities.

Johnson, C. L., & Grant, L. A. (1985). *The nursing home in American society.* Baltimore, MD: Johns Hopkins University.

Johnson, M. (1976). That was your life: A biographical approach to later life. In J.M.A. Munnichs & W.J.A. Van der Heuvel (Eds.), *Dependency or interdependency in old age.* The Hague: Martinus Nijhoff.

Kane, R. A., & Kane, R. (1981). *Assessing the elderly: A practical guide to measurement.* Lexington, MA: Lexington.

Kane, R. L., & Kane, R. A. (1980). Alternatives to institutional care of the elderly: Beyond the dichotomy. *The Gerontologist, 20*(3), 249–259.

Kaufman, H. (1973). *Administrative feedback.* Washington, DC: The Brookings Institution.

Kleemeier, R. W. (1954). Moosehaven: Congregate Living in a community of the retired. *American Journal of Sociology, 59*(4), 347–351.

Knight, B., & Walker, D. (1985). Toward a definition of alternatives to institutionalization for the frail elderly. *Gerontologist, 25*(4), 358–363.

Knowlton, J., Clauser, S., & Fatula, J. (1982). Nursing home pre-admission screening: A review of state programs. *Health Care Financing Review, 3*(3), 75–87.

Kochhar, S. (1977). *SSI recipients in domiciliary care facilities: Federally administered optional supplementation.* Social Security Bulletin, 17–28.

Kusserow, R. P. (1982). *Speech to the National Citizens Coalition for Nursing Home Reform, May 18, 1982* (mimeo). Washington, DC.

Lakin, K. C., Bruininks, R. H., & Hauber, F. A. (1982). *Sourcebook on long-term care for developmentally disabled people.* (CRCS Report No. 17). St. Paul, MN: University of Minnesota.

Lammers, W. W., & Klingman, D. (1984). *State policies and the aging: Sources, trends, and options.* Lexington, MA: Lexington.

Lane, L. F. (1981). The nursing home: Weighing investment decisions. *Hospital Financial Management, 35*(5), 30–45.

Lee, P. R. (1980). *The federal government, health policy and the health care of the disadvantaged.* Paper presented to the Commission on Civil Rights, Washington DC.

Lee, P. R., & Benjamin, A. E. (1983). Intergovernmental relations: Historical and contemporary perspectives. In C. L. Estes, R. Newcomer, & Associates, *Fiscal austerity and aging* (pp. 59–81). Beverly Hills, CA: Sage.

Levit, K. R., Lazenby, H., Waldo, D. R., & Davidoff, L. M. (1985). National health expenditures, 1984. *Health Care Financing Review, 7*(1), 1–35.

Liu, K., & Palesch, Y. (1981). The nursing home population: Different perspectives and implications for policy. *Health Care Financing Review, 3*(2), 15–23.

Lowenthal, M. F. (1964). Social isolation and mental illness in old age. *American Sociological Review, 29*, 54–70.

Lowenthal, M. F., & Robinson, B. (1977). Social networks and isolation. In R. H. Binstock & E. Shanas (Eds.), *Handbook of aging and the social sciences* (pp. 432–456). New York: Van Nostrand Reinhold.

Lyles, Y. M. (1986). Impact of Medicare diagnosis-related groups (DRGs) on nursing homes in the Portland, Oregon metropolitan area. *Journal of the American Geriatrics Society, 34*(8), 573–578.

Melick, C. F., & Eysaman, C. O. (1978). A study of former patients placed in private proprietary homes. *Hospital and Community Psychiatry, 29*(9), 587–589.

Mellody, J. F., & White, J. G. (1979). *Service delivery assessment of boarding homes* (Technical Report). Philadelphia, PA: U.S. Department of Health, Education, and Welfare, Office of the Principal Regional Official, DHEW Region III.

Mendelson, M. A. (1974). *Tender loving greed*. New York: Knopf.

Mor, V., Gutkin, C. E., & Sherwood, S. (1985). The cost of residential care homes serving elderly adults. *Journal of Gerontology, 40*(2), 164–171.

Mor, V., Sherwood, S., & Gutkin, C. (1986). A national study of residential care for the aged. *Gerontologist, 26*(4), 405–417.

Moroney, R. M. (1976). *The family and the state: Considerations for social policy*. London: Longman.

Moss, F. E., & Halamandaris, V. J. (1977). *Too old, too sick, too bad*. Germantown, MD: Aspen.

Newcomer, R. J., & Grant, L. A. (1988). *Residential care facilities: Understanding their role and improving their effectiveness* (Policy Paper No. 21[1]). San Francisco, CA: Institute for Health and Aging, University of California, San Francisco.

Newcomer, R. J., M. P. Lawton, and T. Byerts (Eds.). (1986). *Housing an aging society*. New York: Van Nostrand Reinhold.

Newman, E. S., & Sherman, S. R. (1977). A survey of caretakers in adult foster homes. *Gerontologist, 17*(5), 436–439.

O'Connor, J. (1973). *The fiscal crisis of the state*. New York: St. Martin's.

Olson, L. K. (1982). *The political economy of aging*. New York: Columbia University.

Oregon Administrative Rules. (1985). *Administrative Procedures Act * 183–410, 485,490,500*.

Oregon Administrative Rules (Health Division). (1985). *Long term care facilities * 333–23,80,90*.

Oregon Administrative Rules (Department of Human Resources). (1985). *Residential care, treatment, and training facilities * 410–5*.

Oregon Administrative Rules (Senior Services Division). (1985). *Residential care facilities * 411–55*.

Oregon Department of Human Resources. (1987). *Detailed long term care booklet - February, 1987*. Salem, OR: Senior Services Division.

Oregon Housing Agency. (1987). *Status report, July 1, 1987, Multi-Unit Housing Finance Program, Elderly/Disabled Housing Finance Program, Construction Loan Program, Seed Money Program*. Salem, OR: State of Oregon, Oregon Housing Agency.

Oregon Revised Statutes. (1985). *Home health agencies; residential facilities (ORS), Vol. 3A * * 443*.

Oregon State Senate. (1977a). *Committee on Aging & Minority Affairs, Minutes, January 25, 1977*.

Oregon State Senate. (1977b). *Committee on Aging & Minority Affairs, Minutes, February 15, 1977*.

Oregon State Senate. (59th Legislative Assembly). (1977). *Measure Intent Statement, SB 100*.

Packwood, R. (1981). Long-term care: Costs, financing and alternative public and private policy options. *National Journal, 13*(23), 1039–1043.
Page, D., & Muir, T. (1971). *New housing for the elderly*. London, England: Bedford Square Press for the National Corporation for the Care of Old People.
Palmer, H. C. (1983). Domiciliary care: A semantic tangle. In R. J. Vogel & H. C. Palmer (Eds.), *Long-term care*. Washington, DC: Health Care Financing Administration.
Palmore, E. (1976). Total chance of institutionalization among the aged. *Gerontologist, 16*(6), 504–507.
Paringer, L. (1985). Medicaid policy changes in long term care: A framework for assessment. In C. Harrington, R. J. Newcomer, C. L. Estes, & Associates, *Long term care of the elderly: Public policy issues* (pp. 233–250). Beverly Hills: Sage.
Petersen, M., & Baggett, S. (1985, November). *Predictive nursing home preadmission screening instruments*. Paper presented at the 38th meeting of the Gerontological Society of America, New Orleans, LA.
Peterson, G. E., Bovbjerg, R. R., Davis, B. A., Davis, W. G., Durman, E. C., & Bullo, T. A. (1986). *The Reagan block grants: What have we learned?* Washington, DC: The Urban Institute.
Peterson, P. E., Rabe, B. G., & Wong, K. K. (1986). *When federalism works*. Washington, DC: The Brookings Institution.
Pfeiffer, E. (1975). A short portable mental status questionnaire for the assessment of organic brain deficit in elderly patients. *Journal of the American Geriatrics Society, 23*(10), 433–441.
Pfeiffer, E. (1979). A short psychiatric evaluation schedule: A new 15-item monotonic scale indicative of functional psychiatric disorder. In *Bayer-Symposium VIII: Brain function in old age* (pp. 228–236). New York: Springer.
Pollak, W. (1979). *Expanding health care benefits for the elderly: Volume 1—long term care*. Washington, DC: The Urban Institute.
Reichstein, K., & Bergofsky, L. (1980). *Case studies of state administered residential care programs in Pennsylvania*. Philadelphia, PA: Horizon House Institute.
Reichstein, K., & Bergofsky, L. (1983). Domiciliary care facilities for adults: An analysis of state regulations. *Research on Aging, 5*(1), 25–43.
Rein, M. (1983). *From policy to practice*. Armonk, NY: M. E. Sharpe.
Rice, D. P. (1985). Health care needs of the elderly. In C. Harrington, R. J. Newcomer, C. L. Estes, & Associates. *Long-term care of the elderly: Public policy issues* (pp. 41–66). Beverly Hills, CA: Sage.
Rice, D. P., & Feldman, J. J. (1983). Living longer in the United States: Demographic changes and health needs of the elderly. *Milbank Memorial Fund Quarterly/Health and Society, 61*(3), 362–396.
Risdorfer, E., Primanis, G., & Dozoretz, L. (1971). Family care as a useful alternative to the long-term hospital confinement of geropsychiatric patients. *Journal of the American Geriatrics Society, 19*(2), 150–158.
Roberts, P. (1974). Human warehouses: a boarding home study. *American Journal of Public Health, 64*(3), 277–282.
Rogers, D. E. (1984). Providing medical care to the elderly and poor: A serious problem for the downsizing 1980's. In D. Yaggy (Ed.), *Health care for the poor and elderly: Meeting the challenge* (pp. 3–12). Durham, NC: Duke University.

Rose, A. M., & Peterson, W. A. (Eds.). (1965). *Older people and their social world.* Philadelphia, PA: Davis.

Saul, S. R. (1969). A study of family factors relating to application to a home for the aged (Doctoral dissertation, Columbia University, 1960). *Dissertation Abstracts International, 29*(7), 237A.

Scanlon, W. J. (1980a). Nursing home utilization patterns: implications for policy. *Journal of Health Politics Policy and Law, 4*(4), 619–641.

Scanlon, W. J. (1980b). A theory of the nursing home market. *Inquiry, 17*(1), 25–41.

Schneider, M. (1976). Small group home projects for the elderly. *Journal of Jewish Communal Service, 58*, 88–92.

Segal, S. P., & Aviram, U. (1978). *The mentally ill in community-based sheltered care: A study of community care and social integration.* New York: John Wiley & Sons.

Shanas, E. (1979). Social myth as hypothesis: The case of the family relations of old people. *Gerontologist, 19*(1), 3–9.

Sherwood, C. C., & Seltzer, M. M. (1980, November). *A comparison of state regulations for board and care homes for the elderly, the retarded, and the mentally ill.* Paper presented at the 33rd Annual Scientific Meeting of the Gerontological Society, San Diego, CA.

Sherwood, C. C., & Seltzer, M. M. (1981). *Task III report—Board and care literature review: Evaluation of board and care homes.* Boston, MA: Boston University, School of Social Work.

Sherwood, C. C., & Seltzer, M. M. (1983). *Board and care for the elderly and mentally disabled populations: Final report—Volume IV: A review of the literature.* Denver, CO: Denver Research Institute.

Sherwood, S. (Ed.). (1975). *Long-term care: A handbook for researchers, planners, and providers.* New York: Spectrum.

Sherwood, S., & Gruenberg, M. (1977). *Preliminary analysis of states' licensing requirements for domiciliary care facilities.* Boston, MA: Hebrew Rehabilitation Center for the Aged. (Unpublished).

Sherwood, S., Morris, J. N., & Barnhart, E. (1975). Developing a system for assigning individuals into an appropriate residential setting. *Journal of Gerontology, 30*(3), 331–342.

Sherwood, S., Morris, J. N., & Sherwood, C. C. (1986). Supportive living arrangements and their consequences. In R. J. Newcomer, M. P. Lawton, & T. O. Byerts (Eds.), *Housing an aging society: Issues, alternatives, and policy* (pp. 104–115). New York: Van Nostrand Reinhold.

Soloman, C. D. (1982). *Board and care homes and the Keys Amendment.* Washington, DC: Congressional Research Service, The Library of Congress, Education and Public Welfare Division.

Solon, J., Roberts, D. W., Kruger, D. E., & Baney, A. M. (1957). *Nursing homes, their patients and their care* (PHS Pub. No. 503). Washington, DC: U.S. Government Printing Office.

Sorkin, A. L. (1986). *Health care and the changing economic environment.* Lexington, MA: Lexington.

Starr, P. (1982). *The social transformation of medicine.* New York: Basic Books.

Stassen, M., & Holahan, J. (1981). Long term care demonstration projects: A review of recent evaluations (Working Paper 1227-02). Washington, DC: The Urban Institute.

Stoller, E. P., & Earl, L. L. (1983). Help with activities of everyday life: Sources of support for the noninstitutionalized elderly. *Gerontologist, 23*(1), 64–70.
Stone, D. A. (1984). *The disabled state*. Philadelphia, PA: Temple University.
Stone, R., & Newcomer, R. J. (1986). Board-and-care housing and the role of state governments. In R. J. Newcomer, M. P. Lawton, & T. O. Byerts (Eds.), *Housing an aging society: Issues, alternatives, and policy* (pp. 200–209). New York: Van Nostrand Reinhold.
Stone, R., Newcomer, R. J., & Saunders, M. (1982). *Descriptive analysis of board and care policy trends in the 50 states*. San Francisco, CA: University of California, Aging Health Policy Center.
Swan, J. H., & Harrington, C. (1985). Medicaid nursing home reimbursement policies. In C. Harrington, R. J. Newcomer, C. L. Estes, & Associates, *Long-term care of the elderly: Public policy issues* (pp. 125–151). Beverly Hills, CA: Sage.
Temple University. (1977). *Boarding homes in Philadelphia: Findings, policy implications*. Philadelphia, PA: Temple University, Center for Social Policy and Community Development.
Teresi, J., Holmes, M., & Holmes, D. (1982). *Sheltered living environments for the elderly*. New York: Community Research Applications.
Thompson, F. J. (1986). New federalism and health care policy: States and the old questions. *Journal of Health Politics, Policy and Law, 11*(4), 647–669.
Tinker, A. (1977). Can a case be made for special housing? *Municipal Review, 566*, 314–315.
Townsend, P. (1962). *The last refuge: A survey of residential institutions and homes for the aged in England and Wales*. London: Routledge & Kegan Paul.
Townsend, P. (1963). Measuring incapacity for self-care. In R. Williams, C. Tibbets, & W. Donahue (Eds.), *Processes of aging, social and psychological perspectives* (Vol. 2). London: Athone.
Townsend, P. (1965). The effects of family structure on the likelihood of admission to an institution in old age: The application of a general theory. In E. Shanas & G. F. Streib (Eds.), *Social structure and the family: Generational relations*. Englewood Cliffs, NJ: Prentice-Hall.
Townsend, P. (1981). The structured dependency of the elderly: A creation of social policy in the twentieth century. *Aging and Society, 1*(pt. 1), 5–28.
Trela, J. E. (1971). Some political consequences of senior center and other old age group memberships. *Gerontologist, 2*(2), 118–123.
Tunstall, J. (1966). *Old and alone: A sociological study of old people*. London: Routledge & Kegan Paul.
Underwood, J., & Carver, R. (1979). Sheltered housing: How have things gone wrong—what's coming next? *Housing, 15*(3,4,6).
U.S. Administration on Aging (AOA). Office of Program Development. (1981). *The long term care ombudsman program: Development from 1975–1980*. Washington, DC: U.S. Department of Health and Human Services.
U.S. Bureau of the Census. (1983). *Public-use microdata samples technical documentation*. Washington, DC: Data Users Services Division, Bureau of the Census.
U.S. Congress. House of Representatives, Select Committee on Aging. (1981a). *Hearing: Fraud and abuse in boarding homes*, June 25, 1981, No. 97–295. Washington, DC: U.S. Government Printing Office.
U.S. Congress. House of Representatives, Select Committee on Aging. (1981b). *Hearing:*

Oversight hearing on enforcement of the Keys Amendment, July 28, 1981. Washington, DC: U.S. Government Printing Office.

U.S. Congress. Senate, Special Committee on Aging, Subcommittee on Long Term Care. (1974). *Nursing home care in the United States: Failure in public policy* (Introductory report and supporting papers). Washington, DC: U.S. Government Printing Office.

U.S. Congressional Budget Office. (1977). *Long-term care for the elderly and disabled* (Budget Issue Paper). Washington, DC: U.S. Government Printing Office.

U.S. Department of Commerce. Bureau of the Census. (1977). *Projections of the total population by age and sex for the United States: Selected years 1980 to 2050.* (Current Population Reports Series P–25, No. 704). Washington, DC: U.S. Government Printing Office.

U.S. Department of Health, Education, and Welfare (DHEW). Office of Human Development Services. Federal Council on Aging. (1978a). *Public policy and the frail elderly.* (DHEW Pub. No. [OHDS] 79–20959. Washington, DC: U.S. Government Printing Office.

U.S. Department of Health, Education, and Welfare. Administration for Public Services Office of Human Development Services. (1978b). *Rules and regulations (HDS-AT–78–3 [APS] Implementing Section 505(d) of P.L. 94–566).* Washington, DC: Federal Register, 43(21), 4016–4024.

U.S. Department of Health and Human Services (DHHS). Federal Council on the Aging (FCOA). (1981a). *The need for long-term care information and issues* (DHHS Pub. No. OHDS 81–20704). Washington, DC: U.S. Government Printing Office.

U.S. Department of Health and Human Services. Health Care Financing Administration (HCFA). (1981b). *Long-term care: Background and future directions.* Discussion Paper. (HCFA No. 81–20047.) Washington, DC: Health Care Financing Administration.

U.S. Department of Health and Human Services. Office of the Inspector General. (1982). *Board and care homes: A study of federal and state actions to safeguard the health and safety of board and care home residents.* Washington, DC: U.S. Department of Health and Human Services.

U.S. Department of Health and Human Services. Office of Human Development Services. (1983, November 30). *Standard setting requirements for medical and non-medical facilities where SSI recipients reside: Final rule* (45-CER Part 1397). Federal Register, 48(231), 54184–54187.

U.S. Department of Health and Human Services. Office of Human Development Services. Administration on Developmental Disabilities. (1983). Board and care coordinating unit. *BCCU Memo*, March, 1983.

U.S. Department of Housing and Urban Development. Office of Policy Development and Research. (1976). *Evaluation of the effectiveness of congregate housing for the elderly.* (Final report prepared by Urban Systems Research and Engineering, Inc., Cambridge, MA). Washington, DC: U.S. Government Printing Office.

U.S. General Accounting Office (GAO). (1979). *Identifying boarding homes housing the needy aged, blind, and disabled: A major step toward resolving a national problem.* (Report to the Congress by the Comptroller General of the U.S.). Washington, DC: U.S. General Accounting Office.

U.S. General Accounting Office. (1981). *Improved knowledge base would be helpful in reaching policy decisions on providing long-term, in-home services for the elderly.*

(Report to the Honorable Pete V. Dominici, U.S. Senate). Washington, DC: U.S. General Accounting Office.

U.S. National Center for Health Statistics (NCHS), and Feller, B. A. (1981a). *Health characteristics of persons with chronic activity limitations, 1979.* In Vital and Health Statistics, Series 10, No. 137 (DHHS Pub. No. PHS 81–1565). Washington, DC: U.S. Government Printing Office.

U.S. National Center for Health Statistics, and Hing, B. (1981b). *Characteristics of home residents' health status and care received: National Nursing Home Survey, United States May–December 1977.* In Vital and Health Statistics, Series 13, No. 51. Washington, DC: U.S. Government Printing Office.

U.S. National Center for Health Statistics, and Bloom, B. (1982a). *Current estimates from the National Health Interview Survey, United States, 1981.* In Vital and Health Statistics, Series 10, No. 141 (DHHS Pub. No. PHS 83–1569). Washington, DC: U.S. Government Printing Office.

U.S. National Center for Health Statistics. (1982b). *Living longer in the United States.* Washington, DC: U.S. Government Printing Office.

U.S. National Center for Health Statistics, and Collins, J. G. (1983). *Physician visits, volume, and interval since last visit, United States, 1980.* In Vital and Health Statistics, Series 10, No. 144 (DHHS Pub. No. PHS 83–1572). Washington, DC: U.S. Government Printing Office.

U.S. Public Law 97–35. (1981). *Omnibus Budget Reconciliation Act (OBRA) of 1981.* Washington, DC: U.S. Government Printing Office.

U.S. Public Law 97–248. (1982). *Tax Equity and Fiscal Responsibility Act (HR 4961).* Provisions Relating to Saving in Health and Income Security Programs, passed by Congress, July 12. Washington, DC: U.S. Government Printing Office.

U.S. Public Law 94–566. (1983). *Social Security Act (as amended).* Washington, DC: U.S. Government Printing Office, Social Security Amendments of April 20, 1983, amended) P.L. 98–81, 97 Stat. 65.

U.S. Public Law 98–21. (1983). *Social Security Act Amendments of 1983, April 20.* Washington, DC: U.S. Government Printing Office.

U.S. Public Law 100–203. (1987). *Omnibus Reconciliation Act of 1987 (OBRA).* Washington, DC: U.S. Government Printing Office.

Vicente, L., Wiley, J. A., & Carrington, R. A. (1979). The risk of institutionalization before death. *Gerontologist, 19*(4), 361–367.

Vladeck, B. D. (1980). *Unloving care: The nursing home tragedy.* New York: Basic Books.

Waldo, D. R., Levit, K. R., & Lazenby, H. (1986). National health expenditures, 1985. *Health Care Financing Review, 8*(1), 1–21.

Watt, N. (1970). Five year follow-up of geriatric chronically ill mental patients in foster home care. *Journal of the American Geriatrics Society, 18*(4), 310–316.

Weeden, J. P., Newcomer, R. J., & Byerts, T. O. (1986). Housing and shelter for frail and nonfrail elders: Current options and future directions. In R. J. Newcomer, M. P. Lawton, & T. O. Byerts (Eds.), *Housing an aging society: Issues, alternatives, and policy* (pp. 181–188). New York: Van Nostrand Reinhold.

Weissert, W. G. (1978). Costs of adult day care: A comparison to nursing homes. *Inquiry, 15*(1), 10–19.

Weissert, W., Scanlon, W., Wan, T., & Skinner, D. (1984). Care for the chronically ill: Nursing home incentive payment experiment. *Health Care Financing Review,* 5(2), 41–49.

Zarit, S. H. (1980). *Aging and mental disorders.* New York: Free Press.

Zopf, P. E. (1986). *America's older population.* Houston, TX: Cap & Gown Press.

Index

Activities in daily living (ADL), 16, 123–126
Administrative feedback, 59
Administrative rules, 88–91
Admission/discharge policies, 91–92
Allison, G., 55–56
Alternatives: in areas between organizations, 57; built into goals, 56; requiring coordination, 57
Analysis, 115; descriptive, 116–122; quantitative, 122–128
Assisted living, 143

Bardach, E., 53, 68, 73, 102, 147
Barnhart, E., 108
Bergofsky, L., 45–46
Board and Care Coordinating Unit (BCCU), 75–76
Bovbjerg, R. R., 31
Bradshaw, B., 44
Brody, E., 108
Brody, S. J., 18–19
Brown, L. D., 25, 86–87
Building requirements, 91, 93
Burrows, Mary, 86
Butler, L. H., 7, 9–10, 16

Chronic disease, 17–19
Chubb, J. E., 25

Civil penalties, 84, 86, 142
Coe, M., 28
Community care, 9–10
Conceptual development, 1–11, 79–81
Consensual imperative, 58
"Continuum of care," 5
Corwin, George, 85
Cost containment, 26–29; Medicaid and, 29–31; and reform, 148
Custodialism, 5

Data collection, 111–115
Davis, S. M., 108
Decentralization, 23–25
Demand factors, 21–32
Demographics, 13–15
Department of Health and Human Services (DHHS), 67–70, 75–76
Department of Human Resources (DHR), 82–90; lack of commitment in, 98–99
Descriptive analysis, 116–122
Diagnostic-related groups (DRGs), 27–29
Dick, H., 108
Dunlop, B. D., 61–62

Emergencies, 8–9
Estes, C. L., 2, 7, 14, 24–25, 66, 143

Feder, J., 26, 31, 33
Federal policy, 47–48, 64–77

Index

Feldman, J. J., 15–16
Fire safety, 91
Fiscal crisis, 23–25
Friedsman, H., 108
Funding, 96–97; and quality care, 99–101

Gerard, L., 25
Geriatric Assessment Testing and Evaluation System (GATES) instrument, 110–115, 135
Gibbin, M. J., 108
Goals: alternatives built into, 56; and implementation, 58–59; origins of, 55–56; sequential attention to, 56
Grant, L. A., 42
Gutkin, C., 42, 44, 46

Harrington, C., 23, 30–31, 33
Health care: changing structure of, 21–32; expenditures, 22–23; fiscal crisis and decentralization, 23–25
Health Care Financing Administration, 67
Health care utilization, 17–20
Health, Education, and Welfare (HEW), 72–73
Health Interview Survey (HIS), 15–16
Health services, 92
Health status, 15–17
Hiatt, L., 135
Historical influences, 60–62, 79–81
Holahan, J., 31
Hospital cost containment, 26–29
Housing: need for appropriate, 7; segregated, 8
Hughes, Ted, 86
Hypotheses, 109, 122–128

Imperatives: consensual, 58; legal, 57; national-bureaucratic, 57–58
Implementation, 57–60; administrative rules and Keys Amendment, 88–91; barriers to, 76, 93–94; conceptual areas addressed, 91–92; at the federal level, 70–77; funding and, 99–101; and resources, 59; stages of, 58
Independence, 10–11

Kagan, R. A., 53, 68, 73, 102, 147
Kane, R. A., 54

Kane, R. L., 54
Kaufman, H., 59
Keys Amendment, 51, 64–77; Oregon's experience in implementing, 88–105
Klingman, D., 139
Knight, B., 5

Lammers, W. W., 139
Lane, L. F., 50
Lawson, Charles, 84
Lee, P. R., 2, 14
Legal imperative, 57
Length of stay (LOS), 27
Levit, K. R., 33
Loneliness, 9
Long-term care: demand for, 32–35; and medical model, 1–2; supply factors in, 37–52

Martin, C., 108
Medicaid: advent of, 6; and cost containment, 29–31
Medical model, 102–103; emphasis on, 1–2, 4
Medicare, and hospital cost containment, 26–29
Mental status, 17, 122–123, 126; as critical factor, 133–134
Methodology, 109–115; analysis, 115–128; data collection, 111–115; sample, 110–111
Models of care, 145–146
Morris, J. N., 39, 108
Mor, V., 21, 39–48, 144

National-bureaucratic imperative, 57–58
Newacheck, P. W., 16
Newcomer, R. J., 42
Nixon, R., 65
Nursing homes: alternatives to, 2; early, 49; excessive regulation of, 69; growth of industry, 49–50, 61–62; market for, 50; and Medicaid containment, 30–31; residents of, 19, 131

O'Connor, J., 23
Old Age Assistance (OAA), 60

Older Americans Act (OAA), 2–3; underpinning of, 5
Older people: demographics of, 13–15; and emergencies, 8–9; health care utilization by, 17–20; health status of, 15–17; independence of, 10–11; and loneliness, 9; special needs of, 7–8
Omnibus Reconciliation Act (OBRA), 26, 30–31, 47, 74
Oregon, 79–105; changes of RCF policies and regulations of, 140–144; historical influences in, 79–81; and the Keys Amendment, 88–105
Organizational process paradigm, 55–57
Ownership, 40–42

Paringer, L., 33–34
Patterson, P., 28
Pepper, Claude, 74
Persily, N. A., 18–19
Personnel, 44–45
Policy analysis, 55–62; historical influences on, 60–62; and implementation, 57–60; organizational process paradigm, 55–57
Population characteristics, 15–20
Pugh, Lucille, 85

Quantitative analysis, 122–128

Reform, 139–151; and civil penalties, 142; and costs, 148; models of care, 145–146; the national picture, 144–145; new construction and alterations, 141; of Oregon's RCF policies and regulations, 140–144; role of regulation in, 146–148; services/program/administration, 141–142
Regulations, 53–77; generality of, 132–133; growth of, 53–55; implementation of, 57–60; the Keys Amendment, 64–77; and needs of consumers, 131–137; and policy analysis, 55–63; role of, 146–148
Regulatory unreasonableness, 68–69, 97–98
Reichstein, K., 45–46
Rein, M., 57–59

Research: discussion, 128–129; hypotheses, 109, 122–128; need for, 107, 148–150; questions addressed by, 108–109. *See also* Methodology
Residential care: conceptual confusion regarding, 1–4; conceptual development of, 4–11; costs of service, 42–43; definitions of, 5–6; demand for alternatives, 13–35; and federal policies, 47–48, 64–77; historical influences on, 60–62; personnel, 44–45; range of choice of, 8; regulation of, 53–77; services provided by, 45–47; state policies, 47–48; technology available for, 43–47; theories, assumptions, and rationales underlying, 6–11
Residential care consumers: and the Key Amendment, 70; needs of, 131–137; potential, 20–21
Residential care industry, 37–42
Residential facilities: agenda for the future of, 139–151; definitions for, 83–84; demand for, 94–95; emerging physical design requirements for, 4; generality of regulations for, 132–133; medical nature of, 102–103; ownership of, 40–42; sanctions for, 84, 86–87; size and structure of, 39–40; staffing of, 92–93, 101–105; supply of, 49–52, 95–99
Residents: activities of, 92; assessment of, 135–136; characteristics of, 107–129; mental status of (*see* Mental Status); rights of, 92
Rice, D. P., 15–16
Richard, John, 86
Rinaldo, Matthew, 73

Sanctions, 84, 86–87
Saul, S. R., 108
Scanlon, W. J., 33–34
Scharpf, Martha, 90–91
Schweiker, Richard, 73–74
Segregated housing, 8
Select Committee on Aging, 73–74
Seltzer, M. M., 38
Senate Bill 100 (SB100) (Oregon), 81–

87; impact of, 94–105; implementation of, 88–94
Services, 45–47
Sherwood, C. C., 38–39
Sherwood, S., 39, 42, 44, 108
Social engineering, 7
Social Security Act (1935), 60; amendments to, 61, 64–77
Social support, 128
Solomon, C. D., 54
Sorkin, A. L., 28
Special needs, 7–8
Staffing requirements, 92–93, 101–105; training, 134–135
State policy, and guideline development process, 87
States: and the Keys Amendment, 64; Medicaid and, 29–31; policy, 47–48, 66
Supplemental Security Income (SSI), 54–55
Supply, 49–52, 95–96; factors affecting, 96–99
Swan, J. H., 33
Swoap, David B., 74
Symbolic interactionism, 6–7

Tax Equity and Fiscal Responsibility Act (TEFRA), 30
Technology, 43–47
Theory, 6–11; and implementation, 57–60; return to, 145–148
Townsend, P., 108
Training, 134–135

Vladeck, B. D., 51, 62

Waldo, D. R., 28
Walker, D., 5
Weissert, W., 20
Wilkinson, A., 28

About the Author

SHARON A. BAGGETT is Research Associate, Institute on Aging, Portland State University, Portland, Oregon. Her publications include numerous studies on gerontology.